Living with Parkinson's Disease

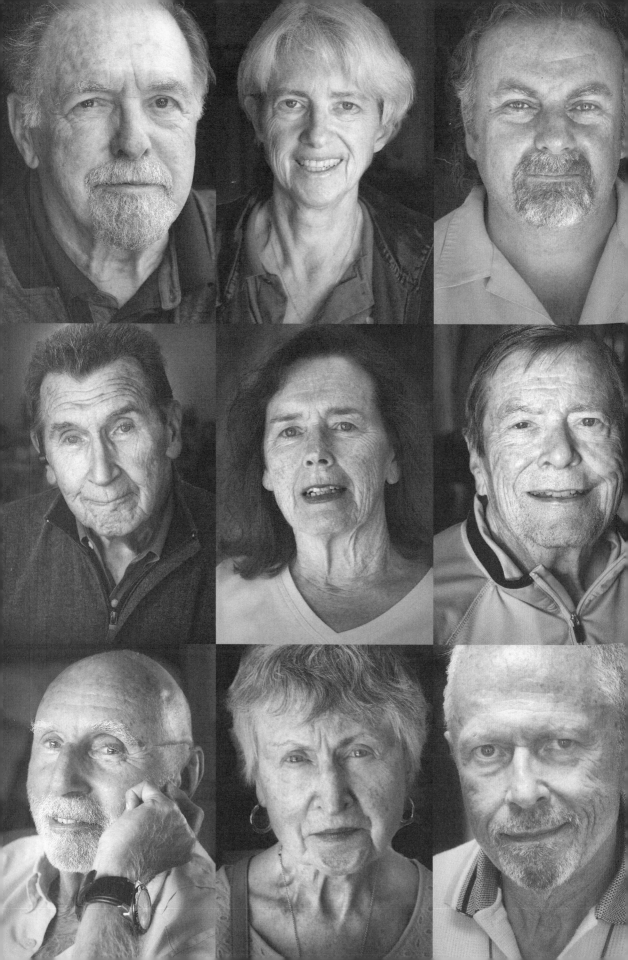

Living with Parkinson's Disease

A COMPLETE GUIDE FOR PATIENTS AND CAREGIVERS

MICHAEL S. OKUN, MD
IRENE A. MALATY, MD
WISSAM DEEB, MD

Robert
ROSE

Design and Production: Kevin Cockburn/PageWave Graphics Inc.
Editor: Johanne Provençal
Copy Editor: Melissa Edwards
Proofreader: Stuart Ross
Indexer: Gillian Watts
Interior Portrait Photography: Bob Dein

Cover image: © gettyimages.com/Grafissimo

Published by Robert Rose Inc.
120 Eglinton Avenue East, Suite 800, Toronto, Ontario, Canada M4P 1E2
Tel: (416) 322-6552 Fax: (416) 322-6936
www.robertrose.ca

Printed and bound in Canada

1 2 3 4 5 6 7 8 9 MI 28 27 26 25 24 23 22 21 20

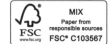

FSC
www.fsc.org

MIX
Paper from
responsible sources
FSC® C103567

This book is dedicated to those persons with Parkinson's disease and their families. Hoping to help you make every day your best day.

CONTENTS

LIVING WITH PARKINSON'S DISEASE

APPENDICES

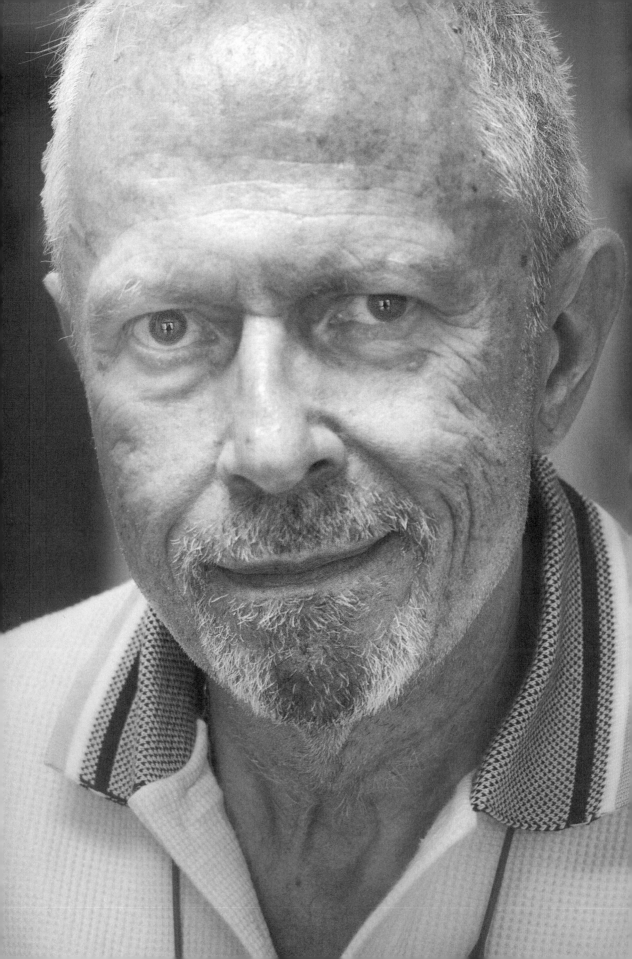

INTRODUCTION

PARKINSON'S DISEASE IS the second most common degenerative disease, trailing only Alzheimer's. Across populations, however, Parkinson's disease is growing at a more rapid rate than Alzheimer's. Due to recent studies, it is now considered undeniable that there is a "Parkinson's pandemic," and as our population survives longer, the burden will expand, stressing patients, families, and the health-care system.

When people hear the words "You have Parkinson's disease," most will envision tragedy. Without interventions, many will spiral into needless demoralization, depression, and despair. But the story does not have to be written in this way. We can teach patients and families from the moment of a diagnosis that Parkinson's disease is a livable condition. It is not Alzheimer's, Lou Gehrig's, or a brain tumor. Parkinson's disease, unlike other neurological conditions, can offer a path to a happier life. There are dozens of effective strategies, including lifestyle changes, medications, surgeries, and other innovative approaches. We have patients who, following the diagnosis of Parkinson's disease, have employed these strategies and tell us their lives are happy and meaningful.

Our first book, *Parkinson's Treatment: 10 Secrets to a Happier Life*, inspired a generation of Parkinson's disease patients and caregivers on their journey to seek meaning and purpose in their lives. One of the secrets from the book was to ask your doctor, at every visit, "What's new in Parkinson's disease?" This inspired a second book, *10 Breakthrough Therapies for Parkinson's Disease*. We have received feedback from all over the world that, while these two books helped many patients and families on the Parkinson's journey, there

The Chinese doctor and philosopher Lu Xun famously said, "Hope is like a road in the country; there was never a road, but when many people walk on it, the road comes into existence." It is critical for us to embrace the current and coming generation of Parkinson's disease patients and to create the path forward. It is important for the Parkinson's patient to understand that there is a road, and that there is a path—a path that includes happiness and fulfillment.

remained a missing, critical element: There was a clear need for practical tips to not just survive the journey, but also to thrive through it.

In this book, as leading Parkinson's disease experts, we have assembled practical tips based on research findings and our own practice as health professionals. Collectively, we have examined thousands of Parkinson's disease patients and written countless prescriptions for medications, surgeries, and rehabilitative therapies. One of us (Okun) has answered more than 20,000 questions on the Parkinson's Foundation website. Over the years, as health professionals specializing in Parkinson's disease, we have experienced both triumph and heartbreak when administering new medication cocktails, experimental drugs, and novel surgical approaches. In this, our third book, we seek to deliver the practical, real-world tips that, when appropriately applied, will enhance the lives of patients and families touched by Parkinson's disease.

The book explores the diagnosis and delves into a deeper understanding of why it is important to understand what you have (i.e., Parkinson's disease) and what you do not have (e.g., Alzheimer's). Unlike previous books, we will discuss in detail rehabilitative therapies, medications for motor and non-motor symptoms, and deep brain stimulation, as well as other innovative surgical approaches. We offer lists, tips, tables, and figures in an effort to summarize the data and make it practical to implement changes into a simple routine. We will address the neglected and exciting areas of nutrition and the microbiome. We also suggest, for readers who are interested in more detailed information, options for further reading throughout the book. Finally, we offer "pearls of wisdom" as well as profiles of heroes who have discovered on their Parkinson's journey that happiness is achievable. We hope you enjoy the practical tips in this book. We believe they have the potential to change lives.

— Michael S. Okun
Irene A. Malaty
Wissam Deeb

SELECTED REFERENCES

Dorsey ER, Sherer T, Okun MS, Bloem BR. The emerging evidence of the Parkinson pandemic. *Journal of Parkinson's Disease*, 2018;8(s1):S3-S8.

Okun MS. *10 Breakthrough Therapies in Parkinson's Disease.* Books4Patients, 2015.

Okun MS. *Parkinson's Treatment: 10 Secrets to a Happier Life.* Books4Patients, 2013.

LIVING WITH PARKINSON'S DISEASE

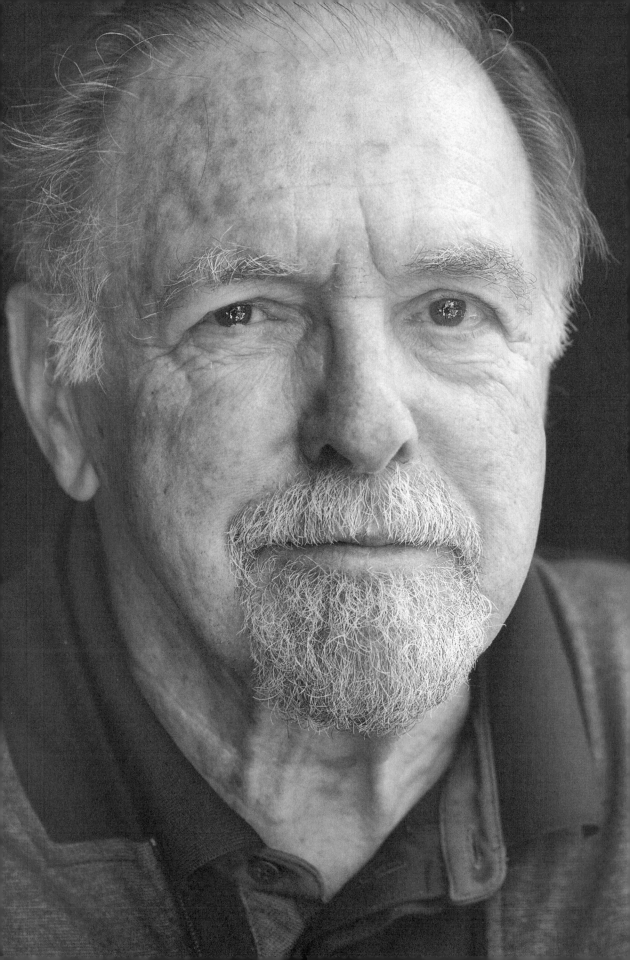

CHAPTER 1

GETTING THE DIAGNOSIS RIGHT

Be sure to put your feet in
the right place, then stand firm.
– Abraham Lincoln

A DIAGNOSIS OF Parkinson's disease can in a moment stun a person and incite fear and bewilderment. Will this change my dreams? What should I do? Who should I tell? Is this serious? The good news is, there is a path to happiness with Parkinson's disease. And the first step should always be to understand what you have and what you do not have.

A common misconception is that Parkinson's disease must have shaking or a tremor. In fact, one in five patients (20 percent) with Parkinson's disease do not have a tremor. Patients and families also tend to have the notion that life is over after a diagnosis of Parkinson's disease. The truth is that Parkinson's patients can live decades and enjoy a meaningful life with appropriate treatment and therapies. It might surprise you to hear that many of our patients tell us their lives are better following the diagnosis of Parkinson's disease, as some discover new talents and others redirect their attention to their health and quality of life. For example, many of our Parkinson's patients who are also CEOs are still working.

Some patients who are diagnosed with Parkinson's disease immediately think of Alzheimer's disease. Their reasoning is simple—they think that "Parkinson's is Alzheimer's with a tremor." Luckily, this could not be further from the truth.

If you receive a diagnosis of Parkinson's disease, you do *not* have:

- Alzheimer's disease
- Lou Gehrig's disease (ALS)
- Multiple sclerosis
- A brain tumor
- A stroke

A few important tips to remember:

◆ Parkinson's disease may or may not have a tremor.

◆ Parkinson's disease patients can live for decades.

◆ Not all Parkinson's disease patients develop memory loss and confusion (and if they develop significant memory issues, it is usually many years down the road).

◆ Parkinson's disease patients, when optimally treated, can enjoy a robust family and personal life.

◆ Many Parkinson's disease patients continue their work lives.

Parkinson's Disease Is Considered a "Clinical Diagnosis"

A clinical diagnosis is:

- Based on the symptoms relayed by the patient and by the examination findings made by the doctor
- Made without a blood test
- Made without a blood pressure cuff
- Made without imaging scans such as a computed tomography (CT) scan or a magnetic resonance imaging (MRI) scan

How Is Parkinson's Disease Diagnosed?

The following features aid in the diagnosis of Parkinson's disease:

- Careful discussion of the symptoms
- An understanding of the changes having an impact on normal daily activities
- Information about the time course and how quickly or slowly symptoms have occurred and/or evolved
- The observations of a trained examiner
- Bedside tests that can help rule out other diseases that may look similar
- Response to dopamine medications over time (carbidopa/levodopa, dopamine agonists, etc.)

The Core Motor Features of Parkinson's Disease

Although Parkinson's disease can present with different symptoms in individual patients, there are some common symptoms that are frequently helpful to a physician in arriving at an accurate diagnosis. It is important to know that not everyone will have each of these symptoms; however, manifesting bradykinesia (slowness) and at least one other cardinal symptom is a requirement. A cardinal symptom is an important symptom commonly observed in Parkinson's disease.

THE FOUR CARDINAL SYMPTOMS OF PARKINSON'S DISEASE

(T) Tremor

(R) Rigidity

(A) Akinesia/bradykinesia

(P) Postural instability and changes in walking

The mnemonic device "TRAP" has been proposed as a way to remember these four "cardinal" (commonly observed) symptoms of Parkinson's disease.

Tremor

The term "pill rolling" has been used to describe the hand tremor. The term was coined based on the action of a pharmacist manipulating a pill between the thumb and index finger. A tremor can be present with action (e.g., action tremor), but typically in Parkinson's disease, the action tremor is mild and the resting tremor (if present) is the more noticeable.

If you ask a random person on the street about Parkinson's disease, a tremor will likely be the most recognized feature. However, 15 to 20 percent of patients with Parkinson's disease do not have a tremor. The majority of patients with a tremor classically experience "rest tremor." A rest tremor is a regular shaking event that is observed when a limb is not engaged in voluntary activity.

Usually, the Parkinson's disease tremor begins on one side of the body, and there is a persistence of asymmetry, even when the tremor affects the other side of the body. The side of the tremor onset is independent of handedness. This means that a right-handed person could present with tremor of the left or the right hand. A common description would be: "My right thumb started twitching whenever I watched TV." Over time, a tremor can possibly affect one or more of the limbs and/or the jaw.

Rigidity

Rigidity refers to a stiffness of muscle movement. Rigidity is commonly worse on one side of the body and, in early Parkinson's disease, it may be present only on one side of the body. Rigidity is also commonly perceived in the neck, arms, and legs. An individual with Parkinson's disease may describe rigidity as tightness or pulling. A misdiagnosis of "frozen shoulder" is a common occurrence following a consultation with an orthopedist or general doctor. As more symptoms emerge, doctors may discover that a frozen shoulder is actually due to Parkinson's disease.

Akinesia/Bradykinesia

Akinesia/bradykinesia refers to a slowness or impairment of movement. In subtle ways, it can manifest as a gradual realization that ordinary tasks (e.g., showering or dressing) are simply taking too long. Another common report is that a spouse, friend, or partner notices that the other person is not keeping up when walking. In a clinic setting, performing rapid repetitive movements, such as tapping the fingers or the feet, can be used to examine the speed of movement, fatigue of movement, and smoothness of movement. These maneuvers can provide key clues to the potential diagnosis of Parkinson's disease.

Postural Instability

Changes having an impact on walking and balance may be important in the diagnosis of Parkinson's disease, but severe walking and balance issues rarely emerge in the first few years following diagnosis. The most common early changes in walking usually involve decreased arm swing and typically occur on one side of the body. A person may complain that one side of the body seems stiff or feels like it is dragging. Sometimes friends may ask if a person has had a stroke. The problem is not weakness, but instead difficulty with movement and coordination, usually on the more symptomatic side of the body.

Parkinson's disease symptoms may include the slowing of walking pace and shortening of steps. As symptoms progress over time, walking may have the appearance of shuffling.

DID YOU KNOW?

A tremor can be a very aggravating symptom and sometimes an annoyance that stubbornly resists treatment with medications. The good news, however, is that cases of Parkinson's disease that are "tremor predominant"—meaning that tremor is a significant component of the presentation—typically have slower changes over time than those that are more heavily affected by stiffness and changes in manner of walking.

One important tip is to ask your doctor to perform a "pull test" on each visit. The pull test is simple to perform and can be used to track balance function. The patient stands up straight and the doctor approaches from behind. The doctor pulls on the shoulders in a backward direction and instructs the patient to take a step or two backward to try to stop from falling. The doctor can intervene if it appears that the patient is at risk of a fall. The test is usually performed two or three times in a row to orient the patient and to help the patient to expect a tug on the shoulder from the doctor. The number of steps necessary to regain balance (if any) is noted at each visit. This test can help identify fall risk, as the more steps backward a patient needs to regain balance, the higher the fall risk.

The normal "postural reflexes"—the ability to catch oneself and avoid falling—may also be impaired. In mild Parkinson's disease, this may result in tripping on uneven surfaces. Common tasks, such as stepping on and off a curbside, may become difficult, and falling can occur when turning. Over time, Parkinson's disease may also result in a stooped posture and leaning to one side. All of these symptoms can collectively have an impact on balance.

Additional Motor Symptoms and Parkinson's Vocabulary

In addition to the four cardinal Parkinson's disease symptoms (the TRAP symptoms), there are additional symptoms that may also emerge. It can be useful for patients to familiarize themselves with the vocabulary for describing Parkinson's disease symptoms.

Micrographia

This refers to small handwriting, similar to the small steps and small finger taps that a patient may encounter in Parkinson's disease.

Masked Facies

This refers to a decrease in facial expressivity or the appearance of a "poker face," and can be mistaken for a lack of emotion.

Dystonia

In Parkinson's disease, a patient's handwriting often gets smaller and sometimes shakier. It may decrease in size the longer a person writes.

Dystonia is a condition that can occur independent of Parkinson's disease but is also commonly observed in Parkinson's disease. Dystonia involves abnormal muscle activation of multiple muscle groups that typically operate in a coordinated fashion, and may result in painful cramping or pulling and, in some cases, twisted postures. The most common forms of dystonia in Parkinson's disease involve the neck (cervical dystonia) or the feet. Neck dystonia may commonly lead to a tilted posture or to muscle pain with tightness. In some cases, dystonia can cause a wiggling or rolling movement that results in tremor of the head. Foot dystonia in Parkinson's disease patients manifests with toe curling (with or without turning in of the foot) or a downward posture of the ankle.

Dyskinesia

This refers to abnormality or impairment of voluntary movement and most commonly occurs four years or more following the diagnosis of Parkinson's disease. Dyskinesia is often observed when medication is at its peak effect (i.e., an hour or more after it is taken). "Diphasic" or "biphasic" dyskinesia is a rare form of dyskinesia that may occur either as dopamine medication takes effect or as it wears off. Dyskinesia will be discussed further in the medication treatment chapter.

Freezing of Gait

This is a symptom more common in advanced Parkinson's disease and not likely to be observed at Parkinson's disease onset. "Freezing" describes the difficulty of initiating movement. This can take the form of a simple delay in starting to walk, or a "stutter-shake" in the legs when attempting walking, but it most commonly occurs as a difficulty in initiating walking. Certain circumstances can trigger freezing. Walking through doorways, stepping into small spaces (such as elevators or closets), and encountering unexpected obstacles (like another person stepping toward the patient) can trigger freezing. Physical therapists can teach techniques to address freezing, which include counting, marching, or imagining a stepping motion over an imaginary line or another person's foot. There are also devices and cues that may be helpful to break the freeze (see Chapter 2).

YOUNG-ONSET PARKINSON'S DISEASE

Parkinson's disease most commonly presents at the age of 60 or later, but it can occur much earlier in life, and is referred to as "young-onset" Parkinson's disease (YOPD) when it begins before the age of 50 (or, by some definitions, before the age of 40). YOPD accounts for no more than 10 percent of Parkinson's disease cases. It affects younger and therefore usually healthier individuals when compared to later-onset Parkinson's disease. In general, it is associated with slower disease progression.

Dystonia, or abnormal muscle activation, can result in cramps and abnormal postures, and seems to be more common in YOPD (although it also occurs in later-onset Parkinson's disease).

Cases that occur before the age of 20 are referred to as "juvenile" Parkinson's disease. Early and young-onset Parkinson's disease is more likely to have an identifiable genetic cause. Early onset cases are associated with more on-off fluctuations, dystonia, and dyskinesia, and tend to involve less memory loss and fewer mobility issues.

Beyond the Obvious: Parkinson's Disease Non-Motor Symptoms

Most people tend to associate Parkinson's disease with motor features such as a tremor. The "non-motor" symptoms can, however, have a more direct and dramatic effect on quality of life. These symptoms, which may be less visibly noticeable, can sometimes precede the onset of motor symptoms. Patients would benefit from becoming familiar with potential non-motor symptoms associated with Parkinson's disease. Here are some of the most common (in alphabetical order).

Anosmia

This refers to the loss of sense of smell that can occur in Parkinson's disease, often many years before any other obvious symptoms are detectable, and is considered a "clinical biomarker" (meaning, a predictor for at-risk Parkinson's disease). There are many other reasons for loss of smell that may be unrelated to Parkinson's disease, including smoking cigarettes and, possibly, seasonal allergies. Anosmia can have an impact on the ability to taste food, as smell and taste are closely integrated. Medication treatments for Parkinson's disease usually do not help this symptom.

Apathy

Apathy is a loss of motivation or initiative. To quote one of our patients with Parkinson's disease, "My get up and go got up and went!" Although apathy can be seen as part of depression, it can occur in Parkinson's disease without depression. It may arise from changes in the circuits of the brain. Sometimes apathy can interfere with follow-through on exercise and on therapy recommendations, and can have an impact on interpersonal relationships. Scheduling activities and psychological therapies can be helpful to address apathy.

Autonomic Nervous System Issues

Parkinson's disease may contribute to or cause dysautonomia (i.e., an abnormality of the automatic or autonomic nervous system), which means that the part of the nervous system that regulates everyday function (e.g., temperature, appetite, blood pressure) becomes unbalanced. Dysautonomia can affect multiple body systems. In the gut, it can slow digestion and contribute to constipation. In the urinary system, it can contribute to troubles with bladder function. In the cardiovascular system, it can result in fluctuations in blood pressure. Another condition, orthostatic hypotension, leads to a dramatic drop in blood pressure while standing, which can be particularly troublesome after prolonged sitting or lying down, as blood may pool in the peripheral blood vessels. As a result of the pooling of blood, there may be ineffective recirculation shortly after standing.

This constellation of changes may lead to the symptoms of light-headedness, feeling off-balance, or passing out. A drop in blood pressure can also be precipitated by a large meal. Some people with Parkinson's disease may experience general blood pressure dysregulation (i.e., very high readings alternating with very low readings, sometimes only moments apart). These blood pressure fluctuations can be very difficult to manage with medication. Management strategies for these problems are discussed in Chapter 5.

Cognitive Changes

Parkinson's disease may contribute to changes in the speed of cognitive processing (thinking), but, if this occurs, it is usually many years following the diagnosis. These symptoms may include difficulty with recalling a desired word or getting the word off the tip of one's tongue. The cognitive changes typically have an impact on the circuits of the brain that are important for planning and executing goal-directed activities. A person with Parkinson's disease and impairment of these functions may find it hard to plan and to complete tasks. Multitasking is especially troublesome in Parkinson's disease. Dementia can occur in some cases of Parkinson's disease.

Constipation

This is another symptom that precedes the onset of obvious motor changes in Parkinson's disease. Over time, changes in the stretching and contractions of the muscles in the gastrointestinal tract (referred to as "gut motility") can have an impact on medication absorption, as slow or erratic intestinal transit of food may affect how consistently medication is absorbed. Most cases can be managed with increased fluid intake and dietary modifications, and with over-the-counter drugs. In severe cases of gastroparesis (i.e., the stomach not emptying), prescription medication may be necessary.

Depression and Anxiety

Depression and anxiety symptoms may arise in Parkinson's disease, sometimes even before the motor symptoms. The root of depression and anxiety in Parkinson's disease is multifaceted. Of course, the diagnosis itself can bring sadness. Worrying about one's future or confronting new symptoms can also provoke an emotional response. The cause for depression with Parkinson's disease, however, is primarily biological, rather than an emotional response to the disease. Parkinson's disease affects dopamine levels and many other brain chemicals and circuits, including serotonin pathways, which contributes to depression and anxiety. Studies have shown that depression has a major impact on quality of life in Parkinson's disease, perhaps even more of an impact than the movement problems. It is critical to address depression and anxiety (i.e., mood symptoms) related to Parkinson's disease.

Fatigue

Lack of energy or general tiredness is one of the most common Parkinson's disease complaints. Poor sleep, medications, and other medical conditions can all contribute. It is important for a doctor to evaluate for general metabolic factors such as thyroid issues. Sleep studies and medication modification can also be helpful.

Hallucinations or Psychosis

Not everyone with Parkinson's disease will experience these symptoms. In advanced Parkinson's disease, however, these symptoms can occur, and they can also be precipitated by certain medications. Most commonly, a person may report a "sense of presence," meaning that they experience the feeling of someone being in the room. If hallucinations occur, the most common type is visual, and is often non-threatening. For example, a person may think they see someone walk by, and then realize there is no one there (i.e., an illusion). Another illusion would be misinterpretation of one object for another (e.g., thinking a pair of socks is an animal).

In mild cases of psychosis, individuals recognize their eyes and brains are "playing tricks" on them, and they are able to overcome the dysfunction without medications. However, in cases where it is hard for the individual to distinguish hallucinations from reality, or if the hallucinations are not pleasant, there are medications that can be used to reduce or to eliminate the problem. Rarely, hallucinations can affect different senses (e.g., hearing or sense of touch). In some cases, Parkinson's disease can result in delusions, or having beliefs that are not consistent with reality, such as mild distrust or paranoia.

Pain

A majority of people with Parkinson's disease report feeling pain, often the tightening and cramping of muscles, particularly when medications wear off. Other sources of pain, like arthritis, are common in the same age group.

REM Behavior Disorder

Rapid eye movement (REM) sleep is a deep, dreaming stage of sleep, in which physical movement is typically very limited. It is common for those with Parkinson's disease, however, to have flailing limbs in their sleep, and to physically "play out" dreams (sometimes including complex fight scenes). The problem is frequently reported by bed partners, and occasionally can lead to injury if the person with Parkinson's disease falls out of bed. Bed partners also can be injured by the movements.

Restless Legs Syndrome (RLS)

This is a condition where a person feels restless, like he or she cannot get comfortable. Most commonly, a person will convey that the legs hurt or that they feel a "creepy-crawly" sensation. Movements such as getting up and walking around usually improve the symptoms. In mild cases, the symptoms may affect only the legs and may occur at night or after prolonged sitting. In more severe cases, the symptoms can affect other body parts and can start earlier in the day. Medication can be helpful in managing this symptom.

Salivary Function

Parkinson's disease may cause what seems like excessive salivation and drooling of saliva (sialorrhea). This symptom is likely due to a decreased rate of natural reflexive swallowing rather than an increase in saliva production. Alternatively, some people with Parkinson's disease report dry mouth, typically as a side effect of medication.

Sexual Health

Parkinson's can affect sexual function. An example is the erectile dysfunction that can occur in men. Physical fluctuations in Parkinson's disease symptoms can also have an impact on social interactions. Psychological factors are also important, such as recognizing and overcoming concerns about a partner's perceptions of the impact of Parkinson's disease.

Sweating

Excessive sweating may be experienced by many people with Parkinson's disease. In some cases, this can be most likely to occur when medications wear off, such as during overnight periods while sleeping.

Fifty-two-year-old Athena has been experiencing a mild tremor in her right hand when reading in the evening. She also finds that quality sleep is harder to get because of leg cramps. She dismisses these issues initially because she has been under more stress at work. Her husband jokes with her that she is trying to attack him in her sleep because she occasionally kicks or punches while dreaming.

Over several months, a few people close to her notice that her right arm isn't swinging the same as her left arm when she walks, and that she no longer keeps the same pace as the people around her. She makes an appointment with her family doctor, who observes the tremor and a slight change in walking, and refers her to a neurologist for suspected Parkinson's disease.

Athena is evaluated and has normal strength and coordination. However, when she is asked to perform rapid repetitive movements, like finger tapping or heel tapping, she has some mild slowness of movements. Her neurologist notices rigidity (stiffness) when she moves her distal limbs (i.e., ankles and wrists) during testing, and her walking has some shortened steps and a decreased arm swing on one side.

Athena is diagnosed with Parkinson's disease and becomes educated about several symptoms she had not understood were related to the disease. These symptoms include constipation and anxiety. She is counseled on available options for treatment and is advised about the importance of exercise. An initial plan is constructed to address her most important symptoms with medication and rehabilitative therapies. Regular follow-up visits to her neurologist are scheduled.

→ CLINICAL PEARL

Studies have revealed that when care teams convey information, it is often received differently by Parkinson's disease patient and by the caregiver. Bringing a caregiver or care-partner to every visit is critical as it can help bridge and clarify any potential communication gaps. Two sets of ears are better than one!

Conditions That Can Look Similar to Parkinson's Disease

There is a well-known saying that "not everything that looks like a duck is a duck." Some other neurological conditions may present with features that look much like Parkinson's disease. However, with time, the progression of symptoms and response to medication often differentiate Parkinson's disease from other conditions. Recognizing these conditions is important so that appropriate expectations can be developed and appropriate treatment can be provided. The appropriate diagnosis may also determine options for participation in research and clinical trials. Here are some of the conditions with symptoms that are similar to Parkinson's disease (in alphabetical order).

Corticobasal Syndrome (CBS)

This condition may present only on one side of the body (i.e., asymmetrically), as Parkinson's disease does. It is common to see significant uncontrollable muscle contraction (dystonia), fast jerks (myoclonus), and an impaired ability for skilled movements in manipulating objects (e.g., apraxia). Sufferers may not, for example, be able to effectively use a screwdriver or scissors.

Drug-Induced Parkinsonism

Some medications may block dopamine receptors and contribute to a syndrome—referred to as "tardive parkinsonism"—that mimics Parkinson's disease. Tremors, stiffness, slowness, and walking changes may all occur. Identifying the medication exposures, even those from the hospital setting, can help evaluate for this possibility. A DaT scan may be useful for diagnosis (see the "DaT Scans" section later in this chapter). Adjusting or discontinuing medication is a common treatment approach and a multidisciplinary team may be helpful to determine the safest possible drug level(s). When there is a co-existent syndrome, such as bipolar disorder, it may not be possible to completely discontinue the dopamine-blocking medication.

In such cases, use of a drug that blocks dopamine but does not worsen parkinsonism (clozapine, quetiapine, or pimavanserin) may be the best approach.

Functional Neurological Disorder

A "functional" disorder is one in which the brain is structurally normal, but abnormal symptoms (or impaired "function") remain. A functional neurological disorder can occur in individuals who have experienced psychological traumas and for whom psychological distress is converted into physical symptoms. These cases are very complex and merit expert involvement along with multidisciplinary treatment.

Multiple Systems Atrophy (MSA)

This is a condition that may present with stiffness and slowness, like Parkinson's disease, but commonly progresses much faster. MSA may additionally have features of "ataxia," or coordination problems. Abnormality of the automatic or autonomic nervous system (dysautonomia), which can be observed in Parkinson's disease, is common and often more severe, especially in the early stages of MSA. Some cases of MSA respond to dopamine.

Normal Pressure Hydrocephalus (NPH)

This is a condition in which the fluid-filled spaces in the brain, called the ventricles, become enlarged. The enlargement stretches other areas of the brain, and as a result there is dysfunction in walking, moving, thinking, and urinating. Although the presentation of symptoms is distinct from Parkinson's disease, there are overlapping symptoms, and occasionally the two are confused. This condition can be diagnosed by using an MRI scan and a spinal drain. NPH can improve in some cases by using shunt surgery.

Progressive Supranuclear Palsy (PSP)

PSP may mimic Parkinson's disease, but, commonly, significant falls occur within the first two years of the disease, in contrast to Parkinson's disease, where falls usually occur later. PSP sufferers may have severe problems with walking, leading to assistive devices or wheelchairs within the first few years of diagnosis. Also, patients may have difficulty voluntarily moving their eyes, especially in the up and down directions (vertical gaze palsy). They may have trouble with certain activities, such as going up and down stairs. Early falling in the first few years after diagnosis is the most common historical feature in PSP.

Vascular Parkinsonism

A series of small strokes in the brain may result in symptoms that mimic Parkinson's disease. Classically, this syndrome has been described as presenting in a "stepwise" fashion, since each stroke event would be associated with a symptom at a different time. Many people with vascular parkinsonism have trouble walking but do not complain of dysfunction with their arms. It has thus been labeled "lower body parkinsonism." This syndrome should be suspected when a neurological history and examination uncover suggestive features, and also when the diagnosis is supported by brain imaging (e.g., MRI). Treatment is focused on reducing the risk of more strokes and using rehabilitation therapy.

DaT Scans

Parkinson's disease can be diagnosed without imaging in nearly all cases. The diagnosis is based on symptoms experienced by the person, signs detected by the examining physician, and the time course of the symptoms. The response to medication is a useful tool in supporting the diagnosis, as regular—or "idiopathic"—Parkinson's disease responds quickly to medications. There are a few exceptions, such as individuals with very mild symptoms, whose improvements are more subtle. On the other hand, a person with more obvious symptoms will usually see immediate and dramatic improvement. Also, if a tremor is the only symptom, this can have an impact on diagnosis, as it is not always resolved with medication.

There are times, however, when imaging can be helpful to clarify the diagnosis. The DaT scan can help confirm or challenge the diagnosis of Parkinson's disease. The test involves injecting a tracer that binds to the dopamine transporter and forms a pattern. The pattern formed for a person with Parkinson's disease is different from the pattern formed for a person without. No test is 100 percent accurate in distinguishing Parkinson's disease from other diagnoses, so this test has to be interpreted in the context of an individual's case.

DaT Scan Limitations

There are also important limitations to DaT scans. A DaT scan can provide evidence of a neurodegenerative condition, but not precisely which one. It cannot distinguish Parkinson's disease from atypical parkinsonism. A doctor can explain the differences between Parkinson's disease, essential tremor, and drug-induced symptoms that mimic Parkinson's.

A DaT scan does not track disease progression and cannot predict how severe a person's symptoms will become. In summary, a DaT scan is rarely required, especially if a patient is seeing an experienced neurologist for a diagnosis. In select cases, a DaT scan can help make the diagnosis and can also be helpful for individuals who feel the need for concrete "data" to embrace a diagnosis.

→ CLINICAL PEARL

Certain medications should not be taken prior to the DaT scan. Be sure your doctor has reviewed your medications with you if this test is ordered.

Deciding When to Consult a Specialist

Many primary care doctors, especially geriatricians, have at least a basic understanding of Parkinson's disease and may be comfortable delivering the initial diagnosis and initiating management. It is advantageous, if available, to

WHAT DO I NEED TO TELL THE DOCTOR?

Visits with your doctor can be optimized by thinking about the most important concerns in advance. This can save time and help ensure every visit can be used to talk through specific questions and concerns. Here are some tips:

◆ For your initial visit, think about the timeline of symptoms. You may not remember every detail, but having a general sense of the time frame is important. Did the symptoms evolve over months or years?

◆ Tell your doctor about your other medical history and any unusual exposures (such as having a history of welding and/or manganese exposure).

◆ Bring a list of medical problems, surgeries, and medications to the visit.

◆ Tell your doctor about any medications you have tried and the benefits or possible side effects you experienced. Provide details about your dosage, if you can.

◆ Share any important impact of your symptoms on your daily life, especially if you wish to see those addressed. For instance, if you find that buttoning a shirt is particularly problematic, your doctor might suggest an occupational therapist who may be able to help.

◆ If applicable, discuss recent events, such as surgeries and hospitalizations, and the impact they had on your Parkinson's disease symptoms. If you are planning surgery, be sure to discuss with your doctor what medications need to be avoided, and discuss any specific recommendations.

◆ Bring a list of any important questions, so you do not forget to ask.

◆ Finally, let your doctor know if you are interested in local support groups or in research.

seek specialty care to optimize counseling and management and to confirm the diagnosis. There is scientific evidence indicating that patients with Parkinson's disease have a better outcome if they see a neurologist. General neurologists should all be familiar to some degree with Parkinson's disease and may have variable comfort with managing the disease. Movement disorder specialists complete extra training (most commonly one to three years) following a neurology residency and are trained to focus on Parkinson's disease and related conditions. When available, movement disorder specialists typically have more experience in managing the complexities of Parkinson's disease.

Additionally, specialty centers may have more options with regard to participating in research trials and may possibly be more familiar with recent developments and directions in the field. In some situations, a specialist may be able to partner with a local neurologist and can alternate visits, keeping the lines of communication open. Also note that rehabilitative therapists (e.g., physical, occupational, and speech therapists) may have varying levels of experience with Parkinson's patients. Some may be able to offer more specialized and specific advice and interventions, while a therapist less familiar with Parkinson's disease may not have the same awareness of alternative approaches and strategies. It is vitally important to have a trusted team that includes doctors familiar and experienced with Parkinson's disease.

Sharing a Diagnosis

The decision to share the diagnosis with family, friends, or colleagues can be complex and is always a matter of personal preference, and it may shift with time. There is nothing wrong with maintaining privacy. A person would not necessarily feel compelled to report a diagnosis of diabetes, for instance. Sharing the diagnosis can be helpful, however, if doing so alleviates the burden of wondering if others have noticed that something is amiss. For instance, a professional might find that explaining she has Parkinson's disease allows her to ignore any notice of her tremor. Sharing this information may also allow for flexibility with regard to day-to-day expectations and timing. On a personal level, sharing with close, trusted friends and family can help with building a support network. We have found over the years that hiding a diagnosis can lead to stress and anxiety for the majority of people who choose this option.

Support Groups

Support groups can be helpful for a number of reasons. Socially, it is valuable to recognize that you are not alone. After all, there are four to six million people in the world living with Parkinson's disease and the numbers are rapidly climbing, especially as people live longer. Connecting with other people can help prevent social isolation and build a network of support. Furthermore, people with Parkinson's disease can share tips and experiences, potentially helping each other identify the best strategies. Support groups often have expert speakers on relevant topics that can be educational for people living with Parkinson's disease. Some types of support groups focus on common interests or goals, like boxing or dancing. Also, life partners of people with Parkinson's disease often benefit tremendously from connecting with others who share this role. Meeting others who are navigating the same physical and emotional issues can be helpful.

FIND A SUPPORT GROUP THAT SUITS YOU

It is important to find a support group that is compatible with you and that suits your needs. Large age differences and different stages of life can be significant factors in your experience of joining a support group. The energy and personality of the group can also have an impact on its value for you. Overall, your involvement should enhance your knowledge and empower you to better manage the condition. It is important to note, however, that many people still working full-time can find support groups to be emotionally challenging.

A Concluding Note

Parkinson's disease is a condition with many symptoms that can affect both physical movement and neuropsychiatric function. Many symptoms may not be obvious signs of Parkinson's disease, but, in many cases, the symptoms are linked. Working with an experienced health-care team to ensure the correct diagnosis is the first step in moving toward the best life possible.

GETTING THE DIAGNOSIS RIGHT

Live as if you were to die tomorrow.
Learn as if you were to live forever.
— MAHATMA GANDHI

➤ The four words "You have Parkinson's disease" are not a death sentence.

➤ Know what you don't have. Parkinson's disease is not Alzheimer's disease, ALS (Lou Gehrig's), or a brain tumor.

➤ Parkinson's disease patients can possibly live 20, 30, 40, or more years following diagnosis.

➤ Parkinson's disease is not one disease. It is a group of symptoms, and the symptoms can vary widely from patient to patient.

➤ Know your Parkinson's disease subtype (tremor dominant, akinetic rigid, postural-instability gait disorder).

➤ After therapy optimization, many patients with Parkinson's disease will tell us their lives are more meaningful following a diagnosis.

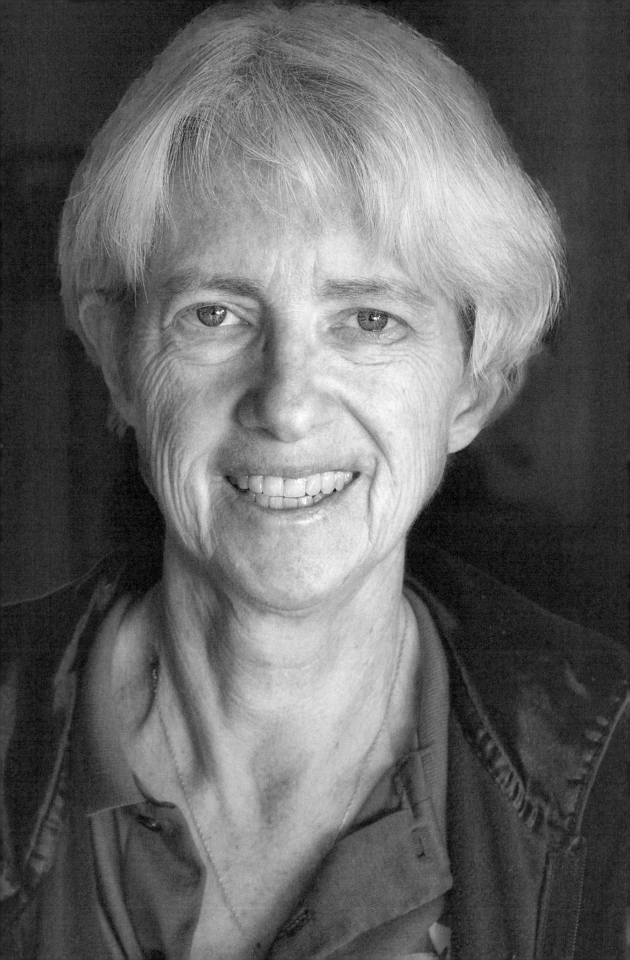

CHAPTER 2

EXERCISE AND REHABILITATION THERAPY

If we could give every individual the right amount of nourishment and exercise, not too little and not too much, we would have found the safest way to health.
– Hippocrates

PARKINSON'S DISEASE AFFECTS multiple body and mind functions. The disease can contribute to multifaceted changes that include motor and non-motor symptoms. Rehabilitation specialists can help manage the symptoms that impact daily function. The team should include physical therapists, occupational therapists, and speech therapists. Health professionals in each of these disciplines can utilize their expertise to manage symptoms such as changes to walking, handwriting, or voice, but they will also work together to formulate a plan to be carried out over time. As the disease progresses, many patients will notice increased challenges with their walking (gait), their balance, and their thinking (cognition). A 2018 study published in *Gait Posture* found that individuals with Parkinson's disease are twice as likely to fall than their peers without Parkinson's disease.

The gait in Parkinson's disease is slow, with small steps, varied speed, and poor control of balance. As the disease progresses, unpredictable changes in walking may emerge, such as freezing of gait (the inability to initiate steps). Freezing can significantly increase the risk of falls and can lead to withdrawal from social activities because of difficulty with walking in the community and a fear of falling. In the early stages of Parkinson's disease, patients can use strategies to compensate for the deterioration in walking. Many therapists encourage exercise to manage challenges with walking and also to decrease the risk of falling. Additionally, if cognition worsens, this compensation may decline as well, and walking may further deteriorate. A 2018 review of 10 years of controlled trials showed that cognitive and gait problems often go hand in hand, and strategies to improve either walking or thinking may actually improve both. In addition, emotions such as anxiety and depression can worsen walking, balance, and freezing events, and potentially contribute to falls. We therefore always recommend addressing other factors, such as thinking and mood, when rehabilitating walking dysfunction.

Doctors often recommend physical, occupational, and speech therapies upon diagnosis of Parkinson's disease, when walking, balance, daily function, and communication are not yet affected. Exercise and rehabilitative therapies are considered first-line approaches to managing Parkinson's disease and a rehabilitation team will assist in treating an individual situation as the condition changes.

In this chapter, we will examine the role of rehabilitation therapies—such as physical therapy, occupational therapy, speech therapy, and other complementary therapies—that may be useful in treating the symptoms of Parkinson's disease, and we will review the evidence for the use of rehabilitative services. Therapy early in the disease has been shown to improve quality-of-life outcomes.

This chapter will answer the following commonly asked questions:

◆ What is rehabilitation?

◆ What is the difference between occupational and physical therapy?

◆ When should I start using rehabilitation services?

◆ What should I expect from my rehabilitation team?

◆ How will these services help me in managing a progressive disease?

The Benefits of Therapy Early On

Knowledge is power when managing Parkinson's disease. Many of the symptoms are very treatable and people can live full lives when provided with the tools to do so early on. Upon diagnosis, it is best for a patient to have a road map, with an understanding of how each provider can help along the way. Physical therapists will help explore a patient's interests in physical activity to determine how to get and keep him or her motivated. It is not good to wait until a patient has physical impairments to start exercising. It is best to stay ahead of the disease. Occupational therapists will help manage a patient's medications, provide coping strategies, and assist with staying engaged in activities, such as work and hobbies. Speech therapists will assist with maintaining voice and social interactions.

CASE EXAMPLE — JULIE

Julie is a 72-year-old woman who lives with her partner in their two-story home. She was diagnosed with Parkinson's disease five years ago. At her current visit with the doctor, she reports that her symptoms have significantly improved since the adjustment of her medications at the previous visit; however, she notes that she is having difficulty taking care of her rose garden. Her partner says that her walking has been changing and she is having episodes of freezing of her steps. On examination, the doctor notices the softening of Julie's voice. The doctor refers Julie for physical, occupational, and speech therapy evaluations.

Frequency of Therapy Visits

Therapists are a critical part of a Parkinson's disease patient's care team. The therapists assist in preventing falls and decline, and help optimize physical and other functions. Therapy should be a part of a patient's life throughout the evolution of the disease, from early to later disease durations. Parkinson's disease is ever-changing and an individual's therapy programs need to change with it. Therefore, it is recommended that a movement disorder therapist be visited at least every six months, so that they can re-evaluate function, compare it to the initial visit, and treat any changes that have occurred. Every six months is a minimum recommendation. If an incident occurs that is having an impact on a person's ability to function successfully—such as a fall, a hospitalization, or a decline in writing—more frequent therapy is warranted to help them return to the previous level of function. Therapy can help an individual complete and "stick to" a plan. If patients lack consistent follow-up, they can struggle with motivation, as mood changes can hinder success with wellness programs. When people see a therapist consistently, they can better address these barriers, such as apathy and lack of motivation.

Beneficial Therapies

Therapists are now specializing in their respective domains. For people with Parkinson's disease, a therapist who works in "neurologic rehab" will best suit their needs. Many patients have had previous experience in therapy to manage orthopedic conditions such as knee pain, back pain, or post-surgical rehabilitation and may have "liked"

TIPS FOR IDENTIFYING A GOOD THERAPIST

To find a good therapist, remember the acronym GOADS:

(G) Goal-directed — Your therapist addresses your needs and provides you with an understanding of what you are trying to achieve together.

(O) One-on-one time — You want to have one-on-one treatments with your provider; your needs will not be met if your therapist is managing two or three patients at the same time.

(A) Anticipation — You look forward to your therapy visits.

(D) Daring — Your visits are challenging.

(S) Support — Your therapist involves your caregivers and support systems in the plan.

---

their therapists, but a complex disorder such as Parkinson's disease is better managed by a neuro-therapist. In addition, there are therapists who specialize in "vestibular" rehab who can treat specific issues related to dizziness and balance. Frequent trips to the bathroom at night can increase fall risk, so seeing a pelvic therapist could help manage bowel and bladder function.

HOW OFTEN DO I NEED TO EXERCISE?

People with Parkinson's disease who exercise earlier in their disease are able to maintain a better quality of life for longer. You need almost 20 minutes per day, which can be done in two 10-minute bouts or one continuous bout. An easy way to get started is to acquire an activity tracker and/or a pedometer to count your steps. Activity trackers can help you determine your baseline levels of activity and help you set goals for the future. Many smart phones can also link to your tracker to provide daily feedback and act as a virtual coach.

Physical Therapy

Physical therapy is also known as physiotherapy. It is a discipline that focuses on using prescribed exercise, manual skills, and patient education to improve the function of an individual suffering from a disease or disease symptom. In Parkinson's disease, a physical therapist (PT) will start by performing a comprehensive evaluation, including tests to examine a patient's strength, flexibility, posture, walking (speed and quality), activity tolerance, coordination, balance, and attention with movement. The PT will then choose the most appropriate therapeutic interventions, with the goal of optimizing mobility for that particular time in the disease process. The PT will discuss exercise protocols, skilled interventions, and fall-prevention strategies, to improve gait, balance, transfers (moving from one position to another), and activity tolerance. The goal of physical therapy will be

THE BENEFITS OF PHYSICAL EXERCISE

Multiple studies have found that physical exercise can significantly improve walking and balance, and, in some cases, can aid in cognition. The benefits of exercise are not limited only to changing the strength and flexibility of the muscles, but can also extend to changes in the brain, positively influencing the brain circuit abnormalities underpinning Parkinson's disease. Doctors treating Parkinson's patients often incorporate exercise into a treatment plan from the time of diagnosis. For those who do not already exercise, starting early in the disease is important, rather than waiting until there is a change in walking or balance. Indeed, many doctors sagely advise using physical exercise as "another medication that you need to take every day." However, for some patients, starting an exercise routine independently can be overwhelming, leaving them feeling like they don't know where to start or what to focus on to ensure they are helping themselves. A physical therapist can help formulate an appropriate exercise routine that provides a safe path for successful management of the disease and for the physical changes that may or may not occur.

to create an individualized treatment plan to improve and maintain independence and increase safety.

Three types of exercise routines exist: aerobic, resistance, and goal-based. Many exercise and physiotherapy training programs for Parkinson's disease combine these and always include a stretching component. Recently, physiotherapists have started using exercise-gaming ("exergaming"), which combines the principles of traditional exercise with an engaging on-monitor or virtual game.

Effect on Thinking (Cognition)

A number of studies have examined the effect of exercise and physical therapy on cognition. Aerobic exercise appears to improve the capacity to inhibit an impulse, to pay attention to the relevant parts of the environment, to multitask, and to deduce, as well as improving reaction time, word finding, and language skills. The evidence for resistance training is limited, but it may improve the capacity to pay attention to "the important things" and to suppress unwanted impulses. Finally, goal-based training in Parkinson's disease, which usually employs something called the "dual-task paradigm," improves the capacity to pay attention to important things, to multitask, and to deduce.

Effect on Emotion

Very few studies have looked into the effect of exercise and physical therapy on emotion in patients with Parkinson's disease. These studies have shown that moderate or treadmill exercise can improve depression.

Effect on Walking (Gait)

Aerobic exercise improves almost all of the components of gait, such as the length of each step, the speed of walking, balance, going up and down stairs, turning, and endurance. Resistance training, in contrast, has provided mixed results, though there seems to be consistent improvements in speed, step length, and balance. Goal-based training improves most of the components of gait, although more studies are needed to clarify the type of goal-based training that may provide the optimal response. The most common strategy to overcome freezing of gait in Parkinson's disease is called "cueing." In cueing, the patient is taught to use either internal cues (e.g., counting) or external cues (e.g., a metronome or visual patterns) to prompt movement. Learning cues can become increasingly difficult with deterioration in thinking (cognitive changes) as the disease progresses. Newer developments, including wearable technology, will help provide automatic "as-needed" cues when the technology senses freezing of gait or other walking problems.

Effect on Posture

Studies have shown that people with Parkinson's disease are able to improve their posture by performing certain exercises (e.g., voluntarily leaning toward an object) and by attempting to control the center of their body as they stand on an unsteady surface (while attached to a safety harness). The improvement in posture can last from weeks to months and may potentially improve balance and reduce falls.

DESIRED EFFECT	CURRENT ROLE OF PHYSICAL THERAPY (AS OF 2019)
Preventing or slowing Parkinson's disease	Experimental
Improving motor symptoms	Good clinical evidence
Treating dyskinesias	Experimental
Improving mood symptoms	Possible

Ongoing Research into Exercise Types

It is not clear if one exercise regimen is superior to others in improving the symptoms in Parkinson's disease. Various published studies have utilized different training programs—for example, the different aerobic exercises featured varying numbers of sessions per week, different times spent in each session, different intensities of exercise, and different types of exercise (e.g., cycling, walking, treadmill). It is also not clear if the stage of Parkinson's disease (early or late) may have a profound influence on the success of the different physical therapy strategies or if the strategies need to be modified according to the stage of the disease. Also, different types of exercises were associated with decreased risk of falls. Strategies that were found to maximally reduce the risk of falls in a 2018 study published in *Gait Posture* included gait training that challenges balance, such as tai chi, a higher amount of exercise (more than 10 hours of exercise per month), and performing most of the sessions under the supervision of a physical therapist. One interesting finding is that people who experience freezing of gait tend to have less improvement and less retention of the skills taught during a training.

In summary, physical therapy improves walking and posture in Parkinson's disease and can decrease the risk of falls. Physical therapy can bring limited improvements to advanced cognitive problems and freezing of gait; posture, however, is more difficult to correct as the disease progresses. Even if the disease is mild, it is important to be

KEY TERMS

Aerobic exercise — Exercises that use a large number of muscles over a period of time (usually 30 minutes or more), with the goal of improving the function of the heart and blood vessels as well as improving general health.

Resistance training — Exercises that use one or a group of muscles by resisting against an external force (such as a weight), with the goal of increasing muscle size, strength, or endurance.

Goal-based/functional training — Exercises that are repetitive and progressive, with the goal of improving a specific set of motor skills; in Parkinson's disease, this is usually accomplished by dual-task training (see next point).

Dual-task training — Exercises that involve doing two exercises at once, such as walking while also performing either a motor or cognitive task (e.g., avoiding obstacles).

Julie arrives at her physical therapy appointment and reports having episodes of sudden inability or hesitation with moving her legs (mainly the left leg), even though she is trying hard to walk. This makes her lose her balance, although she has managed to avoid falling. This freezing is mainly a problem when she is distracted or when turning. It is taking her longer to go up and down stairs.

The physical therapist asks Julie to use a metronome (an instrument that produces a specific sound and steady rhythm) for cueing her steps. As this proves effective, the physical therapist advises Julie to select music with the best rhythm to enhance her walking. The physical therapist also suggests laser shoes or adding contrast to the ground (such as painter's tape on a threshold) to assist Julie with visual cueing of her steps. The physical therapist advises Julie to hold on to the railing at all times when using stairs and to avoid distraction or dual-tasking.

proactive and to initiate a hybrid exercise program supervised by a physical therapist but also including "quasi-independent" activities (such as dance or boxing) or alternative modalities (or approaches to treatment) such as those discussed in later chapters.

The most important components of an effective exercise program include:

◆ High frequency (more than three times per week)

◆ High intensity (bringing heart rate to almost 70 percent of the recommended level for age)

◆ Having more than half of the sessions supervised by a specialized therapist

Having a specialized therapist offers the largest possible advantage, especially with the financial constraints that might limit an intensive program with a physical therapist. The importance of all these components increases as the disease progresses.

Occupational Therapy

Occupational therapy (also known as OT) is a discipline that focuses on using exercise and cognitive-manipulative therapy, through the therapeutic use of daily activities, to improve or to maintain meaningful activities. In Parkinson's disease, OT aims to improve independence in activities at home, at work, and when performing hobbies and other fun activities. Occupational therapy incorporates the caregiver in developing a plan to support the patient's daily activities.

Effect on Daily Activities

Occupational therapy focuses on teaching the person with Parkinson's disease certain strategies to compensate for the limitations that may result from either motor, visual, or cognitive symptoms. These learned skills are helpful in mild cases and continue to help in more advanced cases of Parkinson's disease, especially when paired with the assistance of a caregiver. Some of the strategies include external cues and reminders, appreciating weaknesses and strengths by modifying the task, and increased planning of activities. Planning the day is important in all stages of Parkinson's disease. A study on community re-entry for head-injured adults published in 1987 showed that environmental cueing and adaptation of tasks can be beneficial for ensuring success with daily activities. Occupational therapists have multiple strategies for promoting independence throughout the progression of Parkinson's disease, such as the exploration of adaptive silverware and bathroom modifications.

PLANNING AND PARKINSON'S

Planning your day is cognitively stimulating and can decrease the chances of unforeseen scenarios. Planning also facilitates tailoring your day around fluctuations in medications (and their benefits) and appropriate levels of energy.

Effect on Handwriting

A 2017 study published in the journal *PLoS One* showed that the use of "intensive amplitude training" can improve handwriting in Parkinson's disease. This strategy focuses on increasing the effort of the writing movement while pacing to avoid freezing of movements. The same technique can also improve other daily tasks, such as reaching for objects or putting on a shirt.

Effect on Hand Dexterity

Hand exercise can improve strength and dexterity. People have used different approaches to hand exercise, such as therapeutic putty and coordination training.

Effect on Vision

Visual changes with Parkinson's disease can cause difficulties with daily activities, such as driving, reading, or using a computer. Visual training is a specialized skill in occupational therapy, exploring many strategies to ensure success during these activities. Such strategies include the use of contrast glasses, modifying the environment, and "oculomotor" (eye muscle) training.

Effect on Cognition

Complex daily activities, such as driving or eating in a crowded restaurant, can often prove to be difficult for those living with later stages of Parkinson's disease. Occupational therapists can provide cognitive training and environmental modifications to ensure success with these tasks. As an example, occupational therapists will likely recommend avoiding driving with the radio on, to ensure maximum success and safety.

Effect on the Caregiver

The caregiver in Parkinson's disease plays an important role. The occupational therapist's role extends to ensuring proper education of the caregiver about Parkinson's disease and its requirements, as well as assessing caregiver burden and how to decrease it.

Family Caregiver

Usually a family member who provides physical, emotional, and financial support to a person with a medical condition.

Caregiver Burden

A general term that refers to the "physical, psychological, emotional, social, and financial stresses" experienced by the caregiver as a result of their care duties.

CASE EXAMPLE — JULIE

Julie arrives at her occupational therapy appointment and reports having difficulty taking care of her rose garden, saying it is hard for her to sustain a crouching position and she is easily distracted.

The occupational therapist asks Julie to perform sit-to-stand movements (transfers) daily, increasing the difficulty of the exercise through repetitive standing from progressively lower chair heights to simulate the crouching motion. The occupational therapist suggests that Julie consider using raised gardening beds or an easy-to-move stool to avoid crouching, and to plan frequent breaks to allow for mental and physical recovery. The occupational therapist also advises Julie to plan the steps needed to take care of the garden beforehand, to have them written with easy-to-find cues, and that her partner avoid distracting her by speaking to her when she is gardening. Lastly, the occupational therapist suggests that Julie consider joining a local horticulture group for Parkinson's disease.

Combined Physical Therapy and Occupational Therapy

In most cases, it is advisable to be evaluated by both a physical therapist and an occupational therapist, as they often provide complementary perspectives. For example, both a physical therapist and an occupational therapist will help the patient choose the best assistive device, whether it is a cane, walker, or motorized scooter or wheelchair. A physical therapist will evaluate and adjust the device and tailor it to the patient's needs. An occupational therapist will make sure that there are no obstacles or safety concerns when using these devices at home. It is very important that these assistive devices get tested and adjusted with the supervision of a therapist, as devices that are not properly selected can increase the risk of falls. A full, proper evaluation by a physical therapist and an occupational therapist has been shown to decrease the risk of falling.

Speech Therapy

Speech therapy is also known as speech-language therapy, or SLT. It is provided by a speech-language pathologist (SLP). SLT is a discipline that evaluates speech, swallowing, and language/cognitive impairment, and uses exercises, strategies, and education to improve or maintain function. People with Parkinson's disease commonly develop problems with speech and/or swallowing that can impair their capacity to socialize or participate in meals, difficulties that can result in a decrease in self-confidence or quality of life. These problems are progressive. Speech, swallowing, and language/cognitive function worsen as the disease progresses. There can also be a significant difficulty in word-finding for a number of Parkinson's disease patients.

Effect on Speech

Just like the muscles in the hands, arms, or legs, the muscles that control our ability to speak can be affected by Parkinson's disease. This can cause decreased range of movement in the lips, tongue, and jaw (known as "articulators"), as well as difficulty controlling the voice-box muscles (larynx). This results in an increased rate of speech, often described as short, fast rushes with mumbled words, and/or decreased loudness and changes to voice quality. The natural melody (known as "the prosodic contour") of speech can change as well, leading to monotonous speech. Together, these speech changes are called hypokinetic dysarthria.

One goal of speech-language therapy is to evaluate all the mechanisms involved in speech and identify the best target(s) for therapy. Therapy may consist of exercises and/or implementation of strategies for addressing any speech-related changes. Another goal of speech-language therapy is to improve the loudness and clarity of the voice.

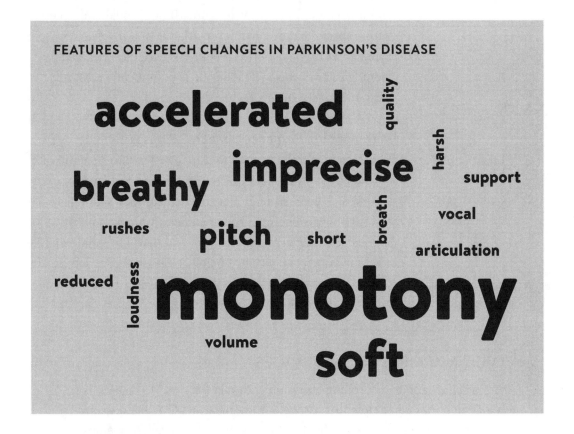

FEATURES OF SPEECH CHANGES IN PARKINSON'S DISEASE

accelerated quality breathy imprecise harsh support rushes pitch short breath vocal reduced loudness articulation monotony volume soft

Some Approaches to Speech Therapy

Lee Silverman Voice Treatment (LSVT)
This is one approach that may improve the loudness of the voice and extend the pitch range. LSVT LOUD (see www.lsvtglobal.com/LSVTLoud) is a speech treatment provided by a certified speech-language pathologist, and involves intensive speech therapy, in one-hour sessions, four days per week for four weeks. The therapy is coupled with daily home exercises to assist with the carry-over of benefits. This is followed by a continuation of home exercises and "tune up" sessions for maintenance of speech benefits.

Expiratory Muscle Strength Training (EMST)

This is an exercise program that aims to increase the strength of the expiratory muscles, which is necessary to exhale air with enough power to produce voice. A commonly researched EMST device is the EMST 150 (see www.emst150.com). EMST involves breathing through a device with a spring-loaded valve for resistance and involves completing five sets of five repetitions, five days per week for at least five weeks. The device is periodically reset as the patient gets stronger.

Maximum Performance Speech Exercises

These are general exercises that may be used to slow the rate of speech, improve clarity of the speech sounds, and increase loudness. A good strategy to use when communicating is SLOP: slow speech rate; speak louder; overarticulate the sounds, making each one distinct; and pause to inhale more air. Individuals can practice using SLOP strategies while reading aloud daily, as this will make it easier to implement in day-to-day conversations.

(S) Slow speech rate

(L) Speak louder

(O) Overarticulate the sounds, making each one distinct

(P) Pause to inhale more air

VOICE AMPLIFICATION DEVICES

Another approach to improving communication in Parkinson's disease is to use a device that can help you improve communication. One inexpensive option is a portable voice amplification device, which several companies sell and which are small enough to fit in a large pocket or small bag. They simply amplify your voice to allow others to hear you more clearly.

Another device option is the SpeechVive (see www.speechvive.com), which fits like an over-the-ear hearing aid. It capitalizes on the "Lombard effect," which is the natural tendency of people to speak louder and slower when there is background noise. The device delivers white noise to your ear, which causes the Lombard effect to trigger louder, slower, and clearer speech. While the SpeechVive is commercially available, it may not be covered by insurance and is more expensive than some of the voice amplification devices. In the U.S., possible funding options for the SpeechVive include insurance reimbursement, reimbursement through the Veteran's Administration (VA), or with a flexible spending account (FSA) or health savings account (HSA).

Effect on Swallowing

Swallowing problems, or dysphagia, are very common in Parkinson's disease. Many people are surprised when these issues are uncovered through testing, as only a minority of patients report such symptoms. Swallowing difficulties place patients with Parkinson's disease at an increased risk for complications such as aspiration (food accidentally entering the airway), leading to aspiration pneumonia, choking, malnutrition, and dehydration. Swallowing problems are a major concern because aspiration pneumonia is the leading cause of death for patients with Parkinson's disease, according to a 2000 study published in *Archives of Neurology*. When swallowing problems occur, symptoms may be obvious, such as increased coughing or even choking on food or liquids, feeling as if the food or pills are stuck in the throat, and possibly unintentional weight loss. However, it is also important to consider that symptoms may be very subtle and go unnoticed, such as feeling a little "tickle" in the neck when drinking or eating, which could be a very small amount of liquid or food going down into the airway. There may not be visual or audible symptoms of swallowing difficulty because swallowing happens quietly and involves structures deep within the neck.

Thus, it is imperative to perform a swallowing evaluation using imaging (called a rehab barium swallow study, modified barium swallow study, or videofluoroscopic swallow study). These types of evaluations allow the speech-language pathologist to view a patient's swallowing as it happens within the neck, by taking X-ray videos while the patient swallows to assess swallowing safety and efficiency. Completing an initial swallow study provides a critical

→ **CLINICAL PEARL**

If you are coughing when eating or drinking, you may be inhaling (aspirating), and a swallowing test would be advisable. A swallowing test consists of swallowing a liquid called barium while a speech therapist examines an X-ray of the action in real time.

baseline to track swallowing changes over time and to be proactive rather than reactive in identifying the best exercises, strategies, and/or diet modifications. Typically, a swallow reassessment is recommended annually.

Many of the throat muscles that are trained during speech therapy play an important role in swallowing. Therefore, many of the exercises that target speech function have positive effects on swallowing. For example, studies have shown that voice training in Parkinson's disease can result in a modest improvement in swallowing and a decrease in the risk of aspiration, and expiratory muscle strength training, biofeedback, and video-assisted training have all shown benefits in decreasing aspiration issues and improving quality of life. In addition, strategies such as changing the position of the head during swallowing, alternating liquids and solids, and changing the bite size are all important and common strategies to decrease swallowing complications.

On rare occasions, patients may require a feeding tube for temporary or permanent means of nutrition, hydration, or consumption of medication. However, it is important to remember that feeding tubes do not eliminate the risk of aspiration issues and they have a significant impact on quality of life. Doctors often advise against feeding tubes for patients with dementia, as they do not significantly extend life expectancy. The decision to use a feeding tube is individual and varies from person to person.

Word-Finding

People with Parkinson's disease may experience increased difficulty finding the words they want to use ("tip of the tongue" phenomenon), which has an impact on their ability to quickly formulate sentences and participate in conversations. Daily tasks that can help with word-retrieval include the following:

- Describing a picture/scene in detail
- Describing each step in a task
- Naming 10 to 20 items in a specific category (e.g., animals, clothing, things that fly, things that are green, words that begin with the same letter, etc.)
- Stating antonyms/synonyms
- Word puzzles (such as crosswords or hangman)
- Word games (such as Scattergories, I Spy, Blurt!, HedBanz, Heads Up!, Pictionary, trivia, etc.)
- Digital applications (such as BrainHQ)

Communication also involves processing, understanding, and using information that is heard or read in an efficient and effective manner. Moreover, since we know that multitasking is more difficult for patients with Parkinson's disease, communicating while completing another simple task (e.g., walking and talking) may prove to be difficult. It is therefore recommended to limit tasks and distractions when focusing on communication.

By describing the object that you are trying to name, you are increasing the connections associated with the "target" word. This may help to retrieve the target word that is on the "tip of your tongue."

A visual aid for word-retrieval strategy, based on a similar diagram in *Community Re-entry for Head Injured Adults* (1987).

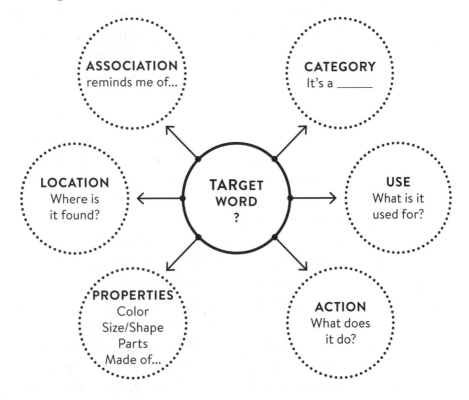

ASSOCIATION reminds me of...

CATEGORY It's a _____

LOCATION Where is it found?

TARGET WORD ?

USE What is it used for?

PROPERTIES Color Size/Shape Parts Made of...

ACTION What does it do?

Other Oral- and Speech-Related Considerations

There are a few additional oral and speech issues that may arise with Parkinson's disease. Here are a few key ones to consider.

Oral Care

Poor oral health strongly correlates with an increased risk of developing aspiration pneumonia. This is because poor oral health results in increased bacteria in the mouth and throat, which, when aspirated with saliva, food, and/or liquids, contributes to increased amounts of bacteria entering the airway and lungs. Interestingly, a 1998 study published in the journal *Dysphagia* found that only 38 percent of known aspirators (with varying medical conditions) developed pneumonia. Oral care should be completed regardless of dental status (natural teeth, dentures, no teeth). Oral care is recommended at a minimum of twice per day, with regular dental appointments every six months.

Dry Mouth

Dry mouth (called xerostomia) is a common side effect of medications. There are limited options for management of dry mouth, including sips of water and products marketed to those with dry mouth (such as Biotène). Furthermore, dry mouth can have a negative impact on oral health, as it can result in increased bacteria production. Therefore, regular oral care should be performed. Use of alcohol-free mouthwash is recommended, as alcohol-based mouthwash can worsen dry mouth and be harsher on the tissues in the mouth.

Extra Saliva/Drooling

Excess saliva (sialorrhea) in patients with Parkinson's disease is thought to be caused by swallowing saliva less frequently (rather than increased saliva production). If too much saliva builds up in the mouth, drooling may occur while upright, or when bending over to complete another task. Conversely, the excess saliva may spill backward into the throat. Drooling can lead to social embarrassment, reduced social participation, and reduced quality of life. Current

Julie arrives at her appointment with her speech-language pathologist and reports that her voice has softened. Her speech-language pathologist engages Julie in speech therapy such as LSVT LOUD and uses other training techniques, such as expiratory muscle strength training (EMST). Julie's speech-language pathologist also informs her that patients with Parkinson's disease are not always aware of swallowing problems and that it is important to evaluate her swallowing when her doctor recommends doing so.

approaches to treatment vary from sensory tricks to medical management. Sensory tricks include hard candy, gum, or sips of water to increase the frequency of swallowing. A doctor should be consulted regarding medication options or more invasive approaches, such as botulinum toxin injections.

Alternative Approaches to Treatment

Multiple nontraditional exercise programs have been developed to improve physical and mental functions in patients with Parkinson's disease. These programs have a common feature—they incorporate standard Parkinson's disease exercise principles into a different and often more enticing environment. For example, the following exercise routines offer balance training (through rapid footwork and whole-body movements, as seen in boxing or dancing), endurance training (through fitness activities), and stretching (through multidimensional movements as well as specific stretching, such as in tai chi), and the use of external cues.

Dance Therapy

Dancing or rhythmic exercise synchronized to music can improve walking, balance, quality of life, and social support in patients with Parkinson's disease. In addition to providing posture-enhancing exercises, balance training, and endurance, dancing provides multiple social and psychological advantages. Several styles of dancing have been shown to be beneficial, such as the tango, waltz, and fox-trot. In addition to helping with walking, dance therapy may improve cognition, motivation, and possibly fatigue. There is growing evidence that traditional and folk dance has a more profound effect, as they activate emotional and memory circuits ("limbic circuits") in the brain. This has been observed with patients engaging in traditional Irish dance, Argentinian tango, and the Sardinian folk dance ballu sardu.

Qigong and Tai Chi

Qigong is a Chinese holistic system that uses meditation, movements, and breathing exercises to rebalance the qi (life energy) and improve health. Tai chi is a martial arts technique that utilizes similar principles to qigong (indeed, many consider tai chi a derivative of qigong) for relaxation through meditation and to strengthen the muscles and body. The exact mechanisms of how qigong or tai chi work on Parkinson's disease remain unknown. The movements are usually gentle and focus on balance and flow. Qigong or tai chi can significantly improve gait and possibly decrease the risk of falls in patients with Parkinson's disease. In addition to helping movement, qigong and tai chi can improve sleep and quality of life.

Acupuncture

Acupuncture is a technique that involves, in all of its forms, the use of hypodermic needles (thin needles inserted through the skin). The needles are applied at specific points across the body, following the concept of life force in traditional Chinese medicine. Acupuncture is thought to rebalance the flow of energy through the body. Variations of traditional, manual acupuncture exist, such as electro-acupuncture (using electrical stimulation) and pharmaco-acupuncture (using bee venom with acupuncture). At the time of writing this book, there is limited evidence that combining acupuncture with regular medication treatments can improve motor function, well-being, and quality of life in patients with Parkinson's disease. Some patients do, however, find acupuncture useful.

WHAT IS THE BEST TYPE OF EXERCISE?

As discussed in this chapter, there are numerous ways to engage in exercise, from indoor to outdoor options, gym programs or group classes, cardiovascular or strengthening, and others. More research is needed to determine which of these is most effective, but the good news is that each has been proven beneficial for people with Parkinson's disease.

Any activity that you engage in daily can help you be successful and prevent decline. All exercise is good exercise and the key is consistency. You need to be more active than sedentary and the more intensely you work, the better the results.

Finally, you are more apt to adhere to your exercise routines when you participate in exercise that you enjoy.

Hydrotherapy

Hydrotherapy refers to the types of exercises that are performed in water (also known as aquatic therapy). This type of therapy offers many advantages over land-based exercises. Most notably, it is safer, as there is a reduced risk of falls. Warm water can also decrease rigidity and stiffness. Studies have shown that hydrotherapy improves gait and mobility in Parkinson's disease to a level greater than what can be achieved by land-based exercises alone. It is important that patients with Parkinson's disease never swim without a partner, as there have been cases of patients freezing up and being unable to move when in the water, leading to a dangerous and life-threatening situation.

Boxing

Many forms of boxing programs for Parkinson's disease are available. These programs combine physical therapy with boxing skills and provide socialization and support. A common boxing program is Rock Steady Boxing. This program includes a multitude of balance, movement, voice, and cognitive exercises to create a comprehensive approach to the symptoms of Parkinson's disease. These boxing programs can improve gait, balance, quality of life, and independence in activities of daily life. As noted for other exercise programs, patients with more advanced Parkinson's disease need more training sessions before they achieve their goals.

Nordic Walking

Nordic walking is a modified walking activity that incorporates the use of poles (similar to ski poles) in both hands. This causes activation not only of the legs, but also of multiple back and arm muscles, producing a higher expenditure of energy. Studies have shown that Nordic walking can help Parkinson's disease symptoms as it improves core strength and posture, enhances endurance, and provides an external cue and rhythm that can improve walking.

Julie reports that she is enjoying her multiple therapies, including physical therapy, occupational therapy, and speech-language therapy. She can tell that her freezing of gait has decreased tremendously and she feels that her balance and confidence in her walking have significantly improved. She has constructed a raised bed for the plants in her garden (although it was somewhat costly), leading to decreased fatigue, and she is enjoying her time with other horticulturists in a Parkinson's disease support group. Her partner has noticed that her voice loudness has improved and that she maintains the benefits of her therapy by persisting with the exercises. Julie reports that when she and her partner went on a trip for three weeks, she did not do her exercises and she noticed that she temporarily lost some of the benefits of her therapies.

A Concluding Note

Physical therapy, occupational therapy, and speech-language therapy are complementary therapies that can significantly improve the movements, the walking (gait), and the quality of life of people with Parkinson's disease. It is important to remember that a one-size-fits-all approach is not effective, and a tailored program involving specialized therapists can provide significant benefits. Many experts are now recommending physical therapy, occupational therapy, and speech-language therapy as first-line therapies, even before physical and voice symptoms emerge.

EXERCISE AND REHABILITATION THERAPY

*All you need is the plan, the road map, and
the courage to press on to your destination.*
— EARL NIGHTINGALE

➻ Not all physical, occupational, and speech/swallow therapy is equal.

➻ Exercise is like a drug for Parkinson's disease. Before there were drugs for Parkinson's disease, exercise was the key.

➻ Rehabilitation therapy (PT, OT, speech/swallow) can be more powerful than drug therapy alone.

➻ Exercise and rehabilitation therapies are now considered first-line therapy for Parkinson's disease.

➻ Be careful taking a prescription for PT, OT, and/or speech/swallow therapy to a therapist who is not trained in Parkinson's disease.

➻ Bad therapy is worse than no therapy.

➻ Occupational therapy is important for reintegrating back into society and back into life.

➻ Speech can be improved by therapy.

➻ If you cough when eating or drinking, you may be at risk for aspiration pneumonia, which is the leading cause of death in Parkinson's disease.

➻ Swallowing issues can also lead to aspiration pneumonia.

➻ There are therapies for improving swallowing and preventing aspiration pneumonia.

➻ Continuous booster therapy (weekly or bimonthly) is superior to burst therapy (e.g., six to eight weeks of intensive therapy, and then done). Spread your rehabilitation therapy visits over an entire year.

➻ Teach a spouse, friend, or personal trainer to direct your home therapy.

SELECTED REFERENCES

Avanzino L, Lagravinese G, Abbruzzese G, Pelosin E. Relationships between gait and emotion in Parkinson's disease: A narrative review. *Gait & Posture*, 2018 Jun;65:57–64. Available at: https://doi.org/10.1016/j.gaitpost.2018.06.171.

Da Silva FC, Iop RDR, De Oliveira LC, Boll AM, De Alvarenga JGS, Filho PJBG, et al. Effects of physical exercise programs on cognitive function in Parkinson's disease patients: a systematic review of randomized controlled trials of the last 10 years. *PLoS One*, 2018;13(2):1–19.

Kulisevsky J, Oliveira L, Fox SH. Update in therapeutic strategies for Parkinson's disease. *Current Opinion in Neurology*, 2018;31(4):439–47.

Langmore SE, Terpenning MS, Schork A, Chen Y, Murray JT, Lopatin D, et al. Predictors of aspiration pneumonia: how important is dysphagia? *Dysphagia*, 1998 Feb;13(2):69–81. Available at: http://link.springer.com/10.1007/PL00009559.

Morgante L, Salemi G, Meneghini F, Di Rosa AE, Epifanio A, Grigoletto F, et al. Parkinson disease survival: a population-based study. *Archives of Neurology*, 2000 Apr;57(4):507–12. Available at: http://www.ncbi.nlm.nih.gov/pubmed/10768625.

Nackaerts E, Broeder S, Pereira MP, Swinnen SP, Vandenberghe W, Nieuwboer A, et al. Handwriting training in Parkinson's disease: a trade-off between size, speed and fluency. Aumann TD, editor. *PLoS One*, 2017 Dec;12(12):e0190223. Available at: http://dx.plos.org/10.1371/journal.pone.0190223.

Paul SS, Dibble LE, Peterson DS. Motor learning in people with Parkinson's disease: implications for fall prevention across the disease spectrum. *Gait & Posture*, 2018 Jan;61:311–9. Available at: https://doi.org/10.1016/j.gaitpost.2018.01.026.

Pinto C, Salazar AP, Marchese RR, Stein C, Pagnussat AS. The effects of hydrotherapy on balance, functional mobility, motor status, and quality of life in patients with Parkinson disease: a systematic review and meta-analysis. *PM&R*, 2019;11(3):278–91.

Pitts T, Bolser D, Rosenbek J, Troche M, Okun MS, Sapienza C. Impact of expiratory muscle strength training on voluntary cough and swallow function in Parkinson disease. *Chest*, 2009 May;135(5):1301–8. Available at: https://linkinghub.elsevier.com/retrieve/pii/S0012369209603111.

Ylvisaker M, Szekeres S, Henry K, Sullivan DM, Wheeler P. Topics in cognitive rehabilitation therapy: cognitive rehabilitation following traumatic brain injury in children. In: Ylvisaker M, Gobble EMR, editors. *Community Re-entry for Head Injured Adults*. College-Hill Press, 1987: 137–220.

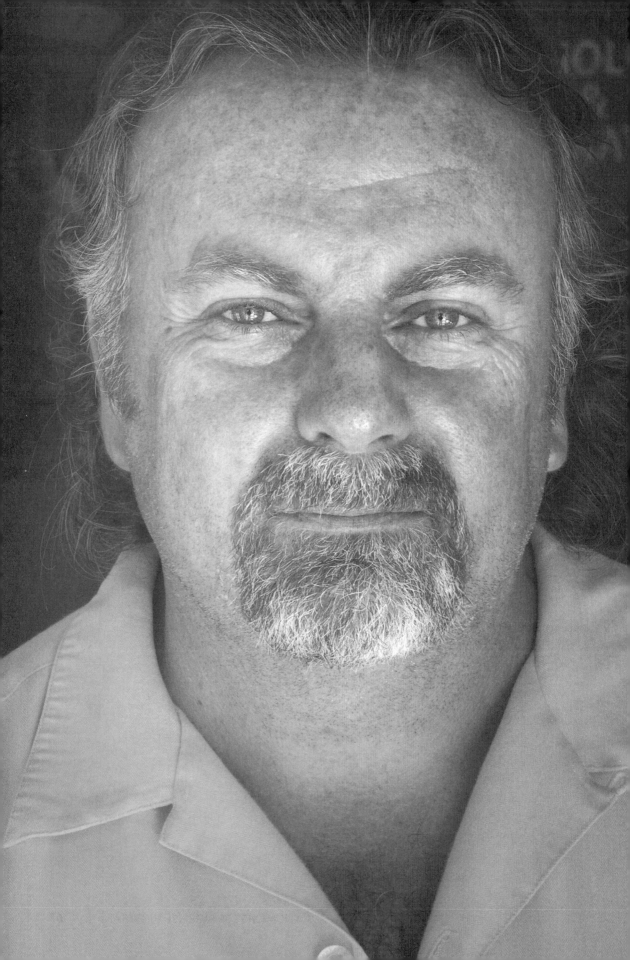

CHAPTER 3

TO START OR NOT START MEDICATIONS FOR PARKINSON'S DISEASE

Start by doing what's necessary;
then do what's possible; and suddenly
you are doing the impossible.
— Francis of Assisi

THE FIRST STEP IN taking control of living a good life with Parkinson's disease is confirming the right diagnosis, processing what the diagnosis actually means, and taking active steps to live the best possible life. This transformation will be different for everyone. For one person, the process can mean continuing work and performing to the level of personal standards. For another, it means being physically active and enjoying travel. Still another individual may use the new diagnosis as an opportunity to change habits and get healthy. All of these goals should be fueled by what works best for each individual to take control of their health and to figure out what it takes to keep doing what makes them who they are.

When it comes to medication, doctors and health-care workers, symposia, reliable websites, and books are all available to help provide information and guidance on the possible medications for use in Parkinson's disease. A more difficult question is, "How and when is the right time for medication?" One obvious sign that medication is appropriate is if there is an impairment in function. We define impairment in function as the loss of the ability to perform tasks, decreasing abilities in a work setting, avoiding social settings, or the presence of physical/emotional issues leading to the loss of enjoyment of physical activity.

The presence of any of these impairments in function signals the need for medication. Common signs of impairment include, for example, noticing a decline in performance at work or difficulty performing physical activities as simple as buttoning a shirt. Sometimes the degree of effort needed to perform the same task becomes increasingly challenging. A more subtle example of impairment would be avoiding a concert or social event because of self-consciousness or the perception that doing so would require excessive effort. In a recent example from our own medical practice, a woman noticed that her husband no longer wanted to accompany her to the grocery store as he had in the past. It is important to remember that when the impact of Parkinson's disease results in a decrease in or withdrawal from activities of daily life, it is important to talk to a doctor about introducing medication.

Another reason to consider medication is to improve quality of life. Although it is not uncommon to be able to perform all daily activities, the presence of Parkinson's disease symptoms, such as a tremor, may result in unnecessary aggravation and have an impact on quality of life. While Parkinson's disease symptoms may not prevent overall functional ability, the aggravation that can come with increased difficulty in performing daily tasks can be a powerful reason to pursue medication.

We have noticed in our medical practices that some professional occupations may be particularly impaired by Parkinson's disease, even when symptoms are only mild. We have evaluated a few trial lawyers and they have conveyed that without medication they cannot be authoritative and compelling in their arguments. Mild slowing of speech, a tremor, or changes in fluidity of movement, for example, have also had an impact on our patients who have frequent public speaking engagements, such as pastors or motivational

Remember, life is multiple choice. Fill your life with the things that bring meaning and enhance your soul with joy and fulfillment. Learning the available options will help put you in the driver's seat. You will then be able to decide if and when to incorporate treatment strategies.

speakers. The reason for the impairment is less important than recognizing that there is an impairment. When the Parkinson's disease symptoms interfere with performing work tasks, enjoying social activities, or participating fully in the activities of daily life, medication has the potential to be the most powerful management strategy, although some patients will try exercise, physical, occupational, and speech therapies first. All of the non-medicinal components are important and they will work together over time to provide different benefits.

Be on the lookout for signs of impairment in function and do not forget that avoiding social settings counts as impairment.

There are also many effective treatments to alleviate other non-motor symptoms, including dizziness on standing, depression, anxiety, apathy, and disorders affecting sleep. Any symptom that results in impairment or is detrimental to well-being should be addressed and medication should be considered. Non-medication approaches, such as the previously mentioned therapies, may be explored first, when appropriate, but medication should be incorporated when the symptoms result in regular or consistent impairment.

CASE EXAMPLE — NICK

Nick is a 68-year-old man who notices a tremor in his right arm when watching television. His wife also observes that his right arm is not moving the same as his left arm while he is walking. Nick has some occasional "catching" of his foot when he walks, but otherwise he isn't really impaired. He describes the issue as "near tripping" and goes to see his doctor to please his wife.

His doctor examines him and finds the strength, reflexes, and sensation in his limbs are normal, but there is some mild stiffness and slowness of movement. He suspects Parkinson's disease and offers Nick treatment options.

Nick holds off on medicine-based treatment because the tremor doesn't bother him initially. He focuses on staying active, as recommended by his doctor, and he has some physical and occupational therapy.

Nine months later, Nick notices his golf game has deteriorated. He continues to work part-time and to function in daily activities without any significant impairment. However, golf is very important to him. He starts a low dose of carbidopa/levodopa (25/100, three times daily) and finds he is better able to have fluid movement and to enjoy walking on the golf course.

Will Medication Cure Parkinson's Disease?

The factors that influence the right time to take medicine may have to do with personal hobbies or unique interests. Discussing pros and cons with your doctor is important.

Medication does not cure Parkinson's disease. Although extensive research is being devoted to slowing disease progression and to discovering a cure, patients should be aware that current therapies do not yet address these gaps. However, current medication can significantly reduce the impact of the symptoms and help those with Parkinson's disease lead a happier and healthier life. Most medication in our cabinets, like blood pressure pills, cholesterol medicine, diabetes medicines, and others, are simply managing the symptoms of a condition and minimizing the impact and suffering that could be associated with the condition. Think of it this way: If blood pressure pills are stopped, the hypertension is still there. But while on the medication, it can be controlled. This is similar to how medication works in Parkinson's disease. The medication generally helps replace or enhance the effect of dopamine and manages the impact of Parkinson's disease. The effects in many cases can be dramatic. There are few medications that have the impact of dopamine replacement.

Prescription Versus Over-The-Counter Supplements

Supplements may not be able to provide the same level of benefits as prescription medication. One supplement, however, does contain levodopa. *Mucuna pruriens*, also known as the velvet bean, is derived from a plant native to Africa and tropical Asia. It has long been used in Ayurvedic medicine to treat Parkinson's disease, but it does not contain carbidopa, so upset stomach can be a concern. In one small 2014 study, published in the journal *Brain*, half of the 14 patients dropped out because of gastrointestinal side effects or worsening motor function with *Mucuna pruriens*, compared to prescription medication, while the other half reported benefits in both mobility and other symptoms of Parkinson's disease.

WHY TAKE MEDICATION?

◆ Impaired function

◆ Symptoms interfere with staying active and engaged

◆ Symptoms are mild but aggravating

◆ Wish to improve quality of life

◆ Mood, sleep, or other non-motor symptoms are detracting from your well-being

In the U.S., supplements are not regulated in the same way as medications, so purity and consistency of contents can vary. Many other supplements, including high-dose Co-Q10 and creatine, have been studied and found in large trials not to be effective in treating the symptoms of Parkinson's disease.

Why Medication Helps

After scientists uncovered the importance of dopamine as a chemical in the brain (known as a "neurotransmitter"), the positive impact of this discovery included significant therapeutic potential (as well as a Nobel Prize). Dopamine is concentrated in the deep areas of the brain referred to as the basal ganglia. Observations in animals have revealed that reduced dopamine or injuries to brain areas that have concentrated levels of dopamine result in symptoms that mimic Parkinson's disease. It was a major development to recognize that replacing dopamine could alleviate many Parkinson's disease symptoms.

→ **CLINICAL PEARL**

Remember that initiating the use of medication does not always mean the use of levodopa and does not always target only motor symptoms.

The drug levodopa was a breakthrough dopamine replacement drug used with Parkinson's disease patients. Levodopa is simply a pill to replace the missing chemical— dopamine—in the brain. This replacement is critical for treating Parkinson's disease. During the early days of dopamine replacement therapy, however, there were challenges in administering medications and also with avoiding extreme side effects, like nausea or vomiting. With further research, doctors realized that adding carbidopa to levodopa resulted in improved outcomes, and many new drugs have since been developed for Parkinson's disease.

There are, for example, dissolving pills for people who have a hard time swallowing, slower-releasing pills, dopamine combined with another medication that helps extend the benefit, inhaled dopamine, and dopamine infused directly into the gastrointestinal tract.

It is worth mentioning that while the dopamine-enhancing medications primarily target motor symptoms, other important symptoms in Parkinson's disease can be addressed with medications that use different mechanisms of action (beyond just dopamine) in an effort to target the non-motor symptoms.

OTHER MEDICATIONS FOR DOPAMINE FUNCTION

There are other medications that work to enhance dopamine function but that use different mechanisms of action. These include dopamine agonists, which activate dopamine receptors; monoamine oxidase type B inhibitors (MAO-B inhibitors); and catechol-O-methyltransferase inhibitors (COMT inhibitors), which slow down dopamine recycling in the brain. There are also other medications with less clear mechanisms of action. These will be further detailed in the next chapter.

Understanding the Controversy over Taking Levodopa

Many years ago, a scientific experiment was published in which levodopa was shown to be "toxic" in cell cultures (in vitro)—when dopamine was added to a dish of cells containing levodopa, the cells were damaged. This experiment contributed to concern that levodopa could be damaging to the dopamine in the brain cells of those with human Parkinson's disease.

This theory has been debunked, because what happens in the human body is not the same as what happens in a dish of cells. In animals and in humans, dopamine replacement has been shown to improve the symptoms, but not to protect against the loss of cells due to the disease itself. Important studies published in the *New England Journal of Medicine* have shown symptomatic but not protective benefits in humans. Neither study supported the false notion that levodopa replacement therapy is toxic.

Some doctors withhold levodopa treatment and some patients refuse treatment, worrying that there will be a toxic effect. This issue has been referred to as "levodopa phobia" and many foundations and experts have published and spoken vigorously to re-educate patients and families about the issue. Levodopa phobia has been propagated through the internet. In addition to levodopa phobia, some patients have personal beliefs or psychological factors that prevent them from taking medications. Some patients erroneously believe that taking medication will lead to disease progression and that the longer they hold out, the better off they will be. In our medical practices, we have observed dozens of tragic cases of levodopa phobia, and in all cases, the patients or doctors withheld medications and a window of opportunity to improve symptoms was lost. In many cases, patients and families express regret and remorse for the "lost years" that were squandered, based on an erroneous belief.

→ CLINICAL PEARL

Here is an insight taken directly from a patient's experience:

I guess I thought I should hold off as long as possible. I heard it was best to do that. I didn't know what I was missing.

Levodopa Phobia and Further Scientific Research

Due to growing interest in any possible destructive effects of levodopa, as well as the potential neuroprotective effects, a study was initiated (and published in the *New England Journal of Medicine* in 2004) to observe if there was any difference between administering levodopa sooner or administering it later. The study also addressed if a lower or higher dose in early levodopa exposure would possibly change the course of the disease. The study—the Early versus Later Levodopa Therapy in Parkinson Disease (ELLDOPA) trial—divided participants into four groups. One group received placebo pills, and the other three groups were administered three different daily doses of levodopa: 150mg, 300mg, or 600mg. At the end of 40 weeks, medication was withheld for two weeks from all participants. The study found that the participants who received levodopa sooner had better scores on scales of Parkinson's disease severity. In fact, the group that received the highest dose benefited the most, and the people who were administered the lower dose treatments still looked better than the placebo group, but not as good as those in a higher dose group. The placebo group had no treatment for 40 weeks. This study suggested that delaying treatment did not help the motor outcomes, and there was no evidence of toxicity. In fact, the treated participants scored better at the end of the study even when off the medication. For this reason, the study also raised the important question of whether levodopa actually slowed the progression of Parkinson's disease.

More than 45 years after levodopa became commercially available, it remains the most effective medication on the market for Parkinson's disease today.

Additionally, in a review published in 1997 in *Parkinsonism & Related Disorders*, more than 800 cases of Parkinson's disease collected over 22 years, pre- and post-levodopa availability, have shown that treatment with levodopa extended the life expectancy of people living with Parkinson's disease. In fact, examining all of the cases of patients with access to levodopa shows that life expectancy was improved by providing earlier treatment. Specifically, people who were treated before developing postural instability seemed to have a greater life expectancy than those who were not treated until progression in their illness to the point of having impaired balance.

Another 2011 study published in *Neurology* examined the outcome from early versus later levodopa treatment and examined the post-mortem brains of 96 people who had had Parkinson's disease. The total lifetime dose of levodopa was compared against markers of disease severity seen under the microscope. The conclusion of the study was that levodopa does not cause progression of Parkinson's disease pathology.

Delays Due to Fear of Dyskinesia

It matters less whether you choose levodopa or a dopamine agonist or another option as first-line therapy. What matters more is that the dose and timing of dosages are optimized to achieve optimal symptom control with minimal or no side effects.

There has been an important question as to whether delaying levodopa could prevent dyskinesia (abnormality of movement resulting in dance-like movements). A few studies have compared outcomes when initiating treatment with levodopa versus different Parkinson's disease medications. One study in 2009, known as the CALM-PD study, compared the outcomes of pramipexole and levodopa as the initial Parkinson's disease medication. Another study compared the outcomes of ropinirole and levodopa. Both of these medications are referred to as dopamine agonists (see Chapter 4). In both studies, the groups starting levodopa later had a longer treatment period before observing dyskinesia, which was initially interpreted (incorrectly) to suggest that dopamine agonists were associated with less dyskinesia. Levodopa is much more potent, however, and therefore demonstrated greater overall improvement in Parkinson's disease symptoms in the study patients. The groups using a dopamine agonist had less overall improvement in symptoms and experienced increased sleepiness.

Dyskinesia is typically observed when therapeutic medication is at its peak benefit and also when dopamine measured in the blood is at its highest concentration. If Parkinson's disease patients are underdosed (meaning they get less than what is needed to control symptoms), dyskinesia is less likely to occur. It is possible that in the original dopamine agonist studies, dyskinesia was less because patients were simply underdosed. Some people interpret these dopamine agonist studies as proving that levodopa should be used rather than the agonist, because it resulted in the most robust motor benefit. Others consider the idea that starting with an agonist may give patients the amount of dopamine needed, and this may be the best strategy for some. This issue is complicated and remains unresolved. In fact, there may be more than one right answer, depending on what matters most to each person, what symptoms are occurring, and what other health factors need to be considered.

There is more evidence that delaying levodopa treatment is not a constructive way to influence dyskinesia onset. A review of medical publications from 1966 to 2000 that studied time to dyskinesia onset found that dyskinesia occurred sooner in patients who had suffered from Parkinson's disease prior to levodopa availability and who ultimately got treated later into their illness. Those patients had sooner onset of dyskinesia, supporting the notion that duration of treatment was not the most important factor. Rather, duration of illness seemed to determine time to onset of dyskinesia. The collective summary of studies was that after four to six years of levodopa treatment, about 40 percent of people experienced some dyskinesia and motor fluctuations. This is discussed further in the next chapter.

How Long Levodopa Works

Many people with Parkinson's disease wonder if there is a lifespan to the benefit that medication can provide. It may help to learn about one 2014 study published in *Movement Disorders*, in which patients were examined over a long period of time to see if they still would benefit from levodopa. The study involved 34 patients who were examined first before starting treatment, then every three years, for an average of 13.3 years (and some up to 20 years). The patients were scored on a motor disability scale (modified Webster scale) while they were both off and on medication. The finding of the study was that improvement from a dose of medication was consistent across time, even when symptom severity increased. Commonly, as the disease changes, the dose required for improvement and the duration of each dose's benefit changes; however, people continue to derive benefit from the medication.

Recent Evidence to Favor Earlier Medication Treatment in Parkinson's Disease

A few recent studies shed new light on early treating and optimizing doses, and suggest that this approach may be justified and preferred. One study compared different geographical populations managing Parkinson's disease in different ways. In parts of Africa, for example, access to levodopa is limited and people commonly cannot obtain medication when desired. Physicians in Africa partnered with physicians in Italy, where levodopa was easily accessed, and the time from diagnosis to treatment was improved. In 2014, a group of 91 Parkinson's disease patients in Ghana was compared to 2,282 Parkinson's disease patients in Italy. On average, levodopa was started two years later in Ghanian patients, so that they got levodopa on average 4.2 years after diagnosis, compared to 2.4 years with the Italian patients.

An important finding emerged from the study: Although both groups had dyskinesia onset six to seven years from the onset of Parkinson's disease, patients from Ghana had dyskinesia at a similar time interval after starting medication. Even when a comparison was made to the Italian patients who did not receive any Parkinson's disease medications other than levodopa, where time to getting levodopa was actually four years sooner than the Ghanians, the time to onset of dyskinesia was the same.

→ CLINICAL PEARL

Dyskinesia is more related to the duration and severity of the disease than it is to the duration of treatment.

A FEW REMINDERS

◆ Assess for impairment in function, meaning the loss of your ability to perform tasks, decreasing abilities in a work setting, avoiding social settings, or the presence of physical/emotional issues leading to impairment of the joy of physical activity.

◆ Starting a medication does not always mean levodopa or a dopamine agonist, as the problem may require treatment for a non-motor issue. Communicating with your health-care team about what symptoms you are experiencing and how they are having an impact on you will help determine when and what treatment is appropriate.

◆ "Winning" is not always avoiding medication. "Winning" is living your best life possible!

The time to onset of dyskinesia did not end up being related to how soon levodopa was started. Instead, what mattered most was how long the person had the disease. The longer someone had Parkinson's disease, the more likely it was that dyskinesia would occur, no matter how long they had been taking levodopa. The study strongly suggested that delaying treatment with levodopa was not effective in delaying or preventing dyskinesia.

In early 2019, the results of another important study were published in the *New England Journal of Medicine*. This was called the Levodopa in Early Parkinson's Disease (LEAP) study. The hope behind this study was to answer the following question once and for all: Does delaying treatment with levodopa provide help or harm in the course of Parkinson's disease? In this study, 445 people in the first few years of the disease were assigned either to delay levodopa treatment as long as possible over the course of 40 weeks (223 patients) or to take levodopa from the start (222 patients) in a random fashion. All participants had similar symptom severity at the beginning and all were treated with levodopa for the second 40-week period of the study (80 weeks in total). After following the outcomes for all 80 weeks of the study, there was neither major benefit nor harm with either group, whether participants were assigned to the early treatment group or to the delayed treatment group. The rates of Parkinson's disease severity and rates of motor complications had no significant differences between early starters of the medication and later starters.

A Concluding Note

The scientific evidence clearly supports that treatment of Parkinson's disease with appropriate medications will improve the symptoms of the disease. Further, alleviating and reducing symptoms helps those with Parkinson's disease stay active in their daily lives. Being active is one of the most important weapons in maintaining physical and cognitive function in Parkinson's disease. It is important to use precisely the amount of medication at an appropriate interval to maintain optimal motor function and quality of life. Patients and families are encouraged to be aware of the research and avoid levodopa phobia. Treatment from medication will not change the speed of disease progression, but it will improve symptoms and offer the best chance for a happier and more meaningful life.

TO START OR NOT START MEDICATIONS FOR PARKINSON'S DISEASE

Start by doing what's necessary; then do what's possible; and suddenly you are doing the impossible.
— FRANCIS OF ASSISI

➻ Do not fall victim to levodopa phobia.

➻ You will not "receive a medal" for delaying therapy.

➻ If Parkinson's disease symptoms are affecting your quality of life or resulting in disability, it is time to start medications.

➻ The hospital is a dangerous place for the Parkinson's disease patient. Every effort should be pursued to avoid hospitalization.

➻ If hospitalized, become your own advocate. You can order an "Aware in Care" hospitalization kit from the Parkinson's Foundation by calling 1-800-473-4636.

SELECTED REFERENCES

Bressman S, Saunders-Pullman R. When to start levodopa therapy for Parkinson's disease. *New England Journal of Medicine*, 2019 Jan;380(4):389–90.

Cilia R, Akpalu A, Sarfo FS, Cham M, Amboni M, Cereda E, Fabbri M, Adjei P, Akassi J, Bonetti A, Pezzoli G. The modern pre-levodopa era of Parkinson's disease: insights into motor complications from sub-Saharan Africa. *Brain*, 2014 Oct;137(Pt 10):2731–42.

Ding C, Ganesvaran G, Alty JE, Clissold BG, McColl CD, Reardon KA, Schiff M, Srikanth V, Kempster PA. Study of levodopa response in Parkinson's disease: observations on rates of motor progression. *Movement Disorders*, 2016 Apr;31(4):589–92.

Fahn S, Oakes D, Shoulson I, Kieburtz K, Rudolph A, Lang A, Olanow CW, Tanner C, Marek K; Parkinson Study Group. Levodopa and the progression of Parkinson's disease. *New England Journal of Medicine*, 2004 Dec;351(24):2498–508.

Parkkinen L, O'Sullivan SS, Kuoppamäki M, Collins C, Kallis C, Holton JL, Williams DR, Revesz T, Lees AJ. Does levodopa accelerate the pathologic process in Parkinson disease brain? *Neurology*, 2011 Oct;77(15):1420–26.

Rajput AH, Uitti RJ, Offord KP. Timely levodopa administration prolongs survival in Parkinson's disease. *Parkinsonism & Related Disorders*, 1997 Nov;3(3):159–65.

Verschuur CVM, Suwijn SR, Boel JA, Post B, Bloem BR, van Hilten JJ, van Laar T, Tissingh G, Munts AG, Deuschl G, Lang AE, Dijkgraaf MGW, de Haan RJ, de Bie RMA; LEAP Study Group. Randomized delayed-start trial of levodopa in Parkinson's disease. *New England Journal of Medicine*, 2019 Jan;380(4):315–24.

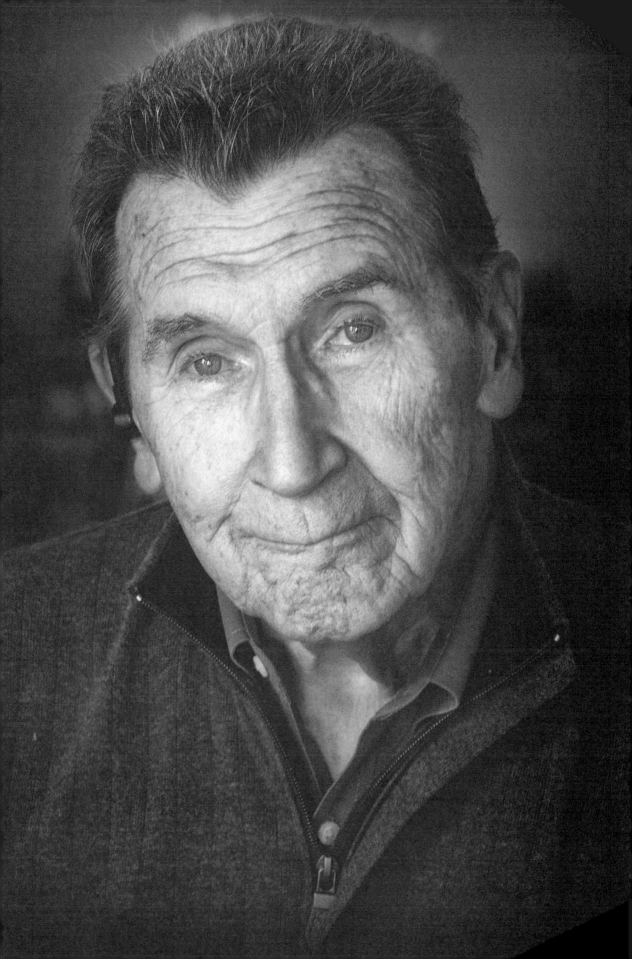

CHAPTER 4

MEDICATION FOR PARKINSON'S DISEASE MOTOR SYMPTOMS

I take the medication for myself so I can transact,
not for anyone else. But I am aware that it is
empowering for people to see what I do.
– Michael J. Fox

PARKINSON'S DISEASE HAS been referred to as the most complex disease in clinical medicine. This is understandable, considering the variety of motor (those that affect movement) and non-motor symptoms, the response to medications, and the use of deep brain stimulation. A few of the most important motor symptoms include tremors (shaking of the hands, usually when resting), slowness of movements, stiffness of the joints (which can result in pain and discomfort), walking changes, poor balance, and falling. In Chapter 3, we reviewed how to make the determination to start medication treatment. In this chapter, we will discuss the different medication options to address the motor symptoms of Parkinson's disease.

The treatment choice should be individualized rather than a standard, one-size-fits-all approach. The reason for individualizing the treatment is the variability of the symptoms of Parkinson's disease, especially over time. Each person with Parkinson's disease possesses a unique combination of symptoms. The choice of medication should ideally target the disability as much as possible. For example, some medications have a strong effect on tremors but a minimal effect on slowness, while others have an excellent effect on both symptoms. Each medication can, however, result in unwanted side effects. The benefits and the side effects vary. Identifying the risks and benefits of each medication is a crucial, initial step in forming the ultimate treatment plan. This risk-and-benefits discussion can be daunting, and some patients will defer to their doctors with statements such as "You know best" or "If you were in my shoes, what would you do?" Others request more information and prefer to review it at their own pace.

A discussion about medication treatment in Parkinson's disease should focus on the following five core principles:

1. What can you expect from the treatment?

2. What are your medication options?

3. What are the symptoms that bother you the most?

4. What can you expect with disease progression?

5. What clinical trials and experimental treatments are relevant?

The information that specialist doctors will provide is derived from the information they have collected through clinical experience and through clinical trials. The longer a medication has been utilized and the larger the number of patients using it, the more confident doctors can be about the benefit-and-risk information. Nonetheless, even with tested medications, there is currently no known way to predict a patient's individual response. Doctors can, however, use some factors to predict a response. For example, the risk of developing the side effect of confusion or hallucinations can be increased by age or in those with preexisting memory problems. However, a trial-and-error process is still usually required until adequate therapy is obtained. Every patient and family should be aware of the need for patience in starting and adjusting Parkinson's disease medication, as it may take weeks to months to realize full benefits.

FINDING INFORMATION ON PARKINSON'S DISEASE MEDICATION

If you are looking for more information, it is important to ensure the quality of the source. Start with your doctor's office, as most will have printed information available for patients that will discuss commonly asked questions and concerns. Patient advocacy organizations, such as the Parkinson's Foundation, the Michael J. Fox Foundation, Parkinson's UK, American Parkinson Disease Association, and the Davis Phinney Foundation, are also useful resources. Pharmacies can provide you with information about your medication; however, not all pharmacists will be equally familiar with the safety of common medications in Parkinson's disease, such as mixtures of monoamine oxidase type B inhibitors (MAO-B) and antidepressants.

Finally, many people commonly access the internet for information, but it is important to pay attention to the parent company (and funding sources) of any website you read, so that you can assess the risk of bias in the information being presented. For example, you may stumble onto a website discussing the management of tremor in Parkinson's disease, but you may also notice either the absence of information regarding the owners of the website or that links on the site bring you to a pharmaceutical company's website. In such cases, when reading the content, keep in mind that the medications made by a particular company may be highlighted at the expense of providing information on other options. In case of doubt, ask your doctor for his or her opinion, or call the Parkinson's Foundation free helpline (1-800-473-4636) to speak to a Parkinson's disease specialist.

COMMON CLASSES OF MEDICATIONS

CLASS OF MEDICATION	EXAMPLES
Levodopa preparations	Carbidopa/levodopa combination (Sinemet) and also benserazide/levodopa (Madopar)
Dopamine agonists	Ropinirole, pramipexole, rotigotine
Monoamine oxidase B (MAO-B) inhibitors	Selegiline, rasagiline, safinamide
Catechol-O-methyltransferase (COMT) inhibitors	Entacapone, tolcapone, opicapone
Others	Trihexyphenidyl, amantadine, istradefylline

Expectations for Medical Treatment

The medications currently available for Parkinson's disease are referred to as symptomatic therapies—they improve the symptoms but do not cure and are not known to affect the course of the disease (although significant research and clinical trials continue to explore ways to alter disease progression). The classification of symptomatic therapy applies to all of the currently available classes of medications that are commonly used to treat Parkinson's disease. The classification also applies to some supplements—two supplements, Co-Q10 and creatine, have been studied in large trials involving Parkinson's disease patients and have not revealed a clear clinical benefit. Conclusions on medications from clinical trials can be complicated, as a clinical trial usually targets one symptom or one outcome, and it could be that a medication failed to address the targeted outcome but did have a different benefit.

The treatments for Parkinson's disease are similar to the treatments for other chronic conditions, such as diabetes. The medications can and, in most cases, will significantly improve the symptoms and quality of life. A significant improvement in the slowness of movements and tremor can be expected, for example. The effect of these medications, which focus on the treatment of motor symptoms (tremor, stiffness, slowness, walking issues, balance), may be less reliable on the non-motor symptoms (such as mood and sleep problems).

Dopamine and the Blood-Brain Barrier

Most of the medication treatments for Parkinson's disease are based on the principle of replacing dopamine. As we discussed in previous chapters, Parkinson's disease symptoms (mainly the motor symptoms) are related to a significant decrease in the brain's production of dopamine. Dopamine is an important chemical for transmitting signals in the brain that are related to the planning and coordinating of movements. In Parkinson's disease, low levels of dopamine may result in slowness and an awkward clumsiness of movements. Since the mid-20th century, scientists have noted that replacing dopamine in the brain can help motor symptoms, including tremor, stiffness, slowness, dystonia, and, in some cases, gait.

The administration of dopamine alone (directly by mouth or as an injection) does not help the motor symptoms because dopamine cannot cross the blood-brain barrier— this is the border that separates the brain from blood and the rest of the body. The blood-brain barrier serves as a block to allow only certain substances to enter the brain, and was designed to protect the brain from infections and other disruptions. In fact, dopamine lingering in the bloodstream can cause severe nausea and vomiting. These limitations triggered the development of different strategies to deliver or increase dopamine in the brain (e.g., adding carbidopa) while at the same time blocking the nausea response.

WHAT IS A CLINICAL TRIAL?

A clinical trial is a type of experiment to test new therapies. In most cases, clinical trials are randomized, double-blind, placebo-controlled studies. This means that there are at least two groups of patients in a study— one receiving the "real" medication and the other receiving an inactive substance with no expected physical effects (called a "placebo"). The patients' allocation to each group is random (randomized) and neither the patient nor the doctor is aware of the group assignments (double blind).

Medications for Parkinson's Disease

What follows is a detailed look at various options for Parkinson's disease medications.

Levodopa

Levodopa, also referred to as L-dopa, remains the most effective medication for the treatment of the general motor symptoms of Parkinson's disease, despite being on the market since the 1970s. Doctors and scientists still refer to this medication as the "gold standard" therapy for Parkinson's disease. Levodopa's ultimate effect is to provide an increase in the amount of dopamine available to the brain. Dopamine cannot cross the highly selective border of the blood-brain barrier; however, levodopa *is* capable of crossing this barrier and so, when taken by mouth or injected, can be transported from the blood into the brain. The brain cells are then capable of transforming levodopa into dopamine. In fact, human brain cells produce levodopa as one of the steps in the natural production of dopamine. This means that levodopa is a precursor or key chemical necessary to producing dopamine. So, taking levodopa provides the brain with a large amount of the precursor it will need to produce dopamine, resulting in an increase in dopamine production in the brain.

HOW CAN I DECIDE ON A MEDICATION?

Choosing a medication can be tricky and stressful and should involve detailed conversation, over time, with your doctor. You and your doctor can review the different available options and assess the risks and benefits of each of these choices, but the discussion should always focus on your particular symptoms. The decision for or against a specific medication is more complex than the simple list of side effects. Your body's reaction to the medication might not match the expected benefit/risk profile for a number of reasons, including your own metabolism and any medical conditions that you have other than Parkinson's disease.

Since levodopa is a form of dopamine, it can get into the bloodstream. Multiple cells in the body outside the brain will transform levodopa into dopamine when they come into contact with it. Intestinal cells, for example, can transform levodopa into dopamine. When levodopa is transformed into dopamine before reaching the brain, it results in nausea and vomiting. Therefore, levodopa is not administered alone, but always in combination with what is called a peripheral decarboxylase inhibitor, which decreases the conversion of levodopa into dopamine in the body and minimizes the risk of nausea.

Levodopa and Peripheral Decarboxylase Inhibitors

When levodopa is transformed into dopamine before reaching the brain, it results in nausea and vomiting. This complication is referred to as "peripheral conversion" (e.g., in the blood) of levodopa to dopamine. Peripheral decarboxylase inhibitors were developed to combat this problem. These substances are combined with levodopa and work only in the rest of the body. Decarboxylase inhibitors cannot cross the blood-brain barrier, but they significantly decrease the conversion of levodopa into dopamine in the body and facilitate more levodopa entering the brain. This also has the benefit of decreasing the risk of nausea and vomiting, since dopamine is not circulating in the blood. The two common combinations include carbidopa/levodopa and benserazide/levodopa (the latter is not approved in the U.S.). Both of these combinations are available in pill form.

MEDICATION DOSAGE AND "HALF-LIFE"

The "half-life" of a medication is the time required for the body to remove half of the administered amount. The half-life is a major determinant of how frequently a medication needs to be taken during the course of a day. Levodopa, as part of carbidopa/levodopa immediate release formulations, has a half-life of 1.5 hours. This means that levodopa requires frequent administrations (at least three times a day). Multiple extended release formulations of levodopa have been developed to prolong this half-life. These extended release formulations either release the medication in a controlled or staggered fashion into the intestines (such as with the brand-name drugs Sinemet CR or Rytary) or in a continuous fashion in the form of an intestinal gel through a feeding-like tube (such as with the brand-name drug Duopa).

When considering the use of a medication, it is essential to consider the duration of effect for each dose, because this will determine how frequently the medication will need to be taken each day. Some medications can be taken once a day, and others are taken multiple times a day. When a drug enters the human body, multiple natural mechanisms attempt to destroy and eliminate it. Each substance is eliminated from the body at a particular speed, and this contributes to how frequently it needs to be taken. Another factor is that the brain cells that convert levodopa to dopamine are also capable of storing the produced dopamine and releasing it at a later time, which may lengthen the effect of the ingested levodopa beyond what is expected. This effect is most pronounced early in the disease progression, when a larger number of cells that can store dopamine are present. As the Parkinson's disease advances, fewer cells that can produce and store dopamine remain and the levodopa therefore needs to be administered more frequently. This has been referred to as the "honeymoon effect," and it can occur early in Parkinson's disease, when patients are noting that a few pills a day are enough to relieve all of their symptoms.

Side Effects of Levodopa

Levodopa is absorbed into the first part of the small intestine by specific transporters that live in the gut and are referred to as "neutral amino acid transporters." These transporters are capable of carrying a specific amount of substances. If more substances are available in the small intestine than can be transported, then the extra amount of these substances will not be absorbed and will be released within the stool. This situation can create a problem when taking levodopa with a heavy meal rich in proteins, thus the usual recommendation to take levodopa at least 30 minutes prior to each meal or to take it two hours after a meal. We will discuss this in more detail in Chapter 7, but for most people, and during most meals, this interaction (which results in decreased levodopa absorption) is negligible and should not be a source of concern.

Tell your neurologist right away about nausea and vomiting, since there are many potential treatments.

The most prominent side effects to consider when using levodopa formulations are nausea and vomiting. It is estimated that up to 20 percent of people develop at least mild nausea when they are first exposed to levodopa. To treat the nausea, we recommend initially taking levodopa with food (as just noted, the interaction of food with levodopa absorption in most instances is not significant). Also, a slow increase in the dose of levodopa is advisable, as nausea usually decreases over time for most people as they

Anti-nausea agents that block dopamine, such as metoclopramide or promethazine, can significantly worsen Parkinson's symptoms (meaning they are contraindicated). Agents such as ondansetron (5HT3 antagonists), trimethobenzamide, or domperidone have all been used successfully with Parkinson's disease. Domperidone, despite being anti-dopamine, works only in the peripheral blood and not in the brain. Thus, domperidone does not have a significant effect at the level of the brain cells and will not worsen Parkinson's disease symptoms.

acclimate to levodopa. In cases where this is not sufficient to alleviate the symptoms, peripheral decarboxylase inhibitors such as carbidopa (in addition to what is already available in the combination pill) is recommended. Using the extended- and controlled-release formulation rather than the usual immediate-release formulations can also be beneficial. Finally, if nausea persists, the addition of anti-nausea medications may be warranted.

Another notable side effect is orthostatic hypotension, which occurs when there is a drop in blood pressure while standing, resulting in a feeling of dizziness, heaviness at the shoulders, or fatigue (when standing up). For most people, the hypotension is temporary and not disabling, but for some, it can be disabling. Ensuring appropriate hydration and salt intake is a must. Further management may require examination and a discussion of treatment options with a neurologist.

Mood and other psychiatric side effects can occur with the use of levodopa. For example, insomnia and anxiety have been reported in about one in every 10 people treated with levodopa. More serious psychiatric side effects, such as hallucinations (seeing things when they are not really there) or delusions (believing irrational thoughts or being paranoid for no credible reason), can occur in less than 5 percent of cases but are more common as the disease progresses. A discussion of the management of these symptoms, which can also occur in Parkinson's disease irrespective of levodopa treatment, is provided in Chapter 8.

A commonly noted side effect is the development of excessive or abnormal movements, or dyskinesias. Studies have shown that the occurrence of dyskinesias is mainly a result of the progression of Parkinson's disease and, to a lesser extent, the dosage and duration of use of levodopa. The prevailing hypothesis is that, as Parkinson's disease progresses, changes in the connections and activations of different brain cells occur that predispose the person to develop excessive movements when exposed to a large amount of externally provided dopamine. Indeed, dyskinesias

DID YOU KNOW?

Some Parkinson's disease patients have trouble with the pill form of medications or must take medications so frequently that a liquid form may be more practical. The table on page 97 provides a common formula to make your own liquid carbidopa/levodopa.

can occur with other agents that increase dopamine, such as dopamine agonists, though at a moderately lower rate. More importantly, delaying treatment with levodopa will not significantly delay the onset of dyskinesia and will not preserve the effect of levodopa in more advanced Parkinson's disease states. The occurrence of levodopa-induced dyskinesias appears to be driven mainly by the duration and progression of the disease. We will discuss the management of dyskinesias and other motor fluctuations later in this chapter.

THINGS TO KNOW ABOUT THE USE OF LEVODOPA

◆ Levodopa is widely considered the gold standard for Parkinson's disease.

◆ Levodopa is not toxic.

◆ Experts recommend taking the amount of levodopa that you need.

◆ The initial use of levodopa is commonly associated with nausea and vomiting.

◆ There are many strategies to manage the possible associated side effects.

Finally, there has been considerable controversy on whether levodopa causes Parkinson's disease to progress faster. As discussed earlier in this book, this concern has its roots in older studies that showed that there was decreased dopamine cell survival when levodopa was added to cells in a petri dish. This type of experiment is artificial and is referred to as "in vitro," meaning they are performed outside the human. Multiple human studies have shed light on the controversy. Levodopa, in humans, does not appear to be toxic and does not result in a faster progression of Parkinson's disease. Experts in Parkinson's disease have largely debunked the myth that levodopa is toxic in humans.

Dopamine Agonists

The term "dopamine agonists" refers to a group of drugs that interact directly with the dopamine receptors located on nerve cells in the brain, which are called "neurons." Neurons process information received from other brain cells or body sensors and communicate by forming a communication channel called a "synapse." This is a small, highly specialized space where the membranes of the two cells are close but do not touch. For example, neuron A will release chemicals, called "neurotransmitters," inside the synapse (the communication channel). The surface of neuron B contains receptors that can receive the information released from the neurotransmitter. One such neurotransmitter is dopamine.

Dopamine agonists work by directly attaching to the dopamine receptors on neuron B, replacing the lost signals from the dying-off of dopamine cells in Parkinson's disease. Thus, the dopamine agonists can improve the symptoms simply by tickling the receptors on neuron B. In addition, dopamine agonists can cross the blood-barrier directly, unlike dopamine.

Three common dopamine agonists are pramipexole, ropinirole, and rotigotine. All of these agents are similarly effective in treating the motor symptoms of Parkinson's disease, either as monotherapy (meaning, this is the only Parkinson's disease drug administered) or in combination with other drugs. Another agent, piribedil, is not available in the U.S. There are other, older dopamine agonists, called "ergot-derived agonists," and these include cabergoline, dihydroergotamine, pergolide, and bromocriptine. These ergot-derived dopamine agonists are efficacious but less

LIQUID LEVODOPA

The following table for liquid levodopa is provided courtesy of and with permission from the Parkinson's Foundation educational series on Parkinson's disease medications:

FORMULA FOR LIQUID SINEMET

1mg levodopa per 1ml solution

- Sinemet, 25/100 tablets, 10 tablets (1000mg levodopa; do not use Sinemet CR)
- Ascorbic acid (vitamin C) crystals, ½ tsp (approx. 2g)
- Tap water or distilled water, 1 liter or 1 quart

1. Mix the above ingredients in a liter/quart plastic container with lid (do not use metal).
2. Rotate or shake gently until tablets dissolve (no need to crush them). Tablets may not go completely into solution.
3. Formula will maintain full strength and purity for 24 to 48 hours in refrigerator.

DOSING RECOMMENDATIONS

Always establish a dosing plan with your physician or health-care provider first!

Morning ("jump start") dose:

- 60ml of the formula (60mg or a little more than ½ of a 25/100 tablet of carbidopa/levodopa) or use amount comparable to usual tablet dose.
- Adjust dose 5–10ml up or down every three to five days until you achieve the best "ON" response with the least dyskinesia.

Hourly dosing:

- 30ml of the formula on the hour while awake or hourly proportion of usual tablet dose (e.g., a person taking one carbidopa/levodopa 25/100 tablet every two hours might try 50ml per hour of the liquid).
- Adjust dose 5–10ml up or down every three to five days until "ON" periods are smoother.

For the best overall result, it is strongly recommended that you adjust the morning "jump start" dose prior to adjusting the hourly doses. Accuracy of the dose and exact hourly timing between doses is critical for optimal benefit. Optimal dosing can vary tremendously from one person to another.

commonly used due to concerns about the development of cardiac and lung complications (scarring of the heart valves and lungs). Dopamine agonists have in many cases been used as monotherapy. Levodopa is also commonly used as monotherapy.

PRONUNCIATION KEY

(stressed syllable in **bold**)

Levodopa	Lee-voe-**doe**-pa
Carbidopa	Car-bee-**doe**-pa
Ropinirole	Row-**pin**-er-ole
Pramipexole	Pram-i-**pex**-ole
Rotigotine	Row-**tig**-oh-teen
Apomorphine	Ae-poe-**more**-feen
Selegiline	Sell-**edge**-ah-leen
Rasagiline	Rah-**saj**-ah-leen

Pramipexole and ropinirole are available as pills (which can be immediate-release or delayed-release). Rotigotine is available in the form of a daily patch. All of the dopamine agonists share similar side effects, most notably excessive sleepiness and sleep attacks, swelling of the ankles, low blood pressure and dizziness when standing up, mood changes, and impulse control disorder (ICD). ICD (e.g., excessive shopping, gambling, hypersexuality, binge eating) can be the most concerning side effect of dopamine agonist use. Levodopa, in contrast, may result in mania (racing thoughts) and/or sexually deviant behavior(s). Both dopamine agonists and levodopa can be associated with the occurrence of "punding," which is the performance of repetitive and often mechanical tasks, such as taking apart a watch and putting it back together. Longer-acting formulations of dopamine agonists—and particularly the patch—have been associated with a lower risk of ICD. When starting dopamine agonists, there should always be a monitoring plan in place in case ICD emerges.

Dopamine Agonist Withdrawal Syndrome

It is important to consult with a doctor when decreasing the use of dopamine agonists, as withdrawals can be disabling (comparable to withdrawal from cocaine). Dopamine agonist withdrawal syndrome (DAWS) can include a combination of symptoms, including depression, confusion, anxiety, suicidal thoughts, lack of motivation, dizziness when standing up, hot flashes, excessive sweating, nausea, vomiting, decreased appetite, fatigue, sleep problems, and even dopamine agonist drug craving. DAWS can happen even with a very slow decrease in the dose of the dopamine agonists. The treatment is to restart the dopamine agonist, even at a smaller dose. Treating the symptoms of DAWS with other agents, such as more levodopa, anxiety medications, antidepressants, nausea medications, or blood pressure medications, is not effective. The only improvement that may occur for a small proportion of patients is when the dopamine agonist is restarted.

THINGS TO KNOW ABOUT THE USE OF DOPAMINE AGONISTS

◆ Experts no longer uniformly recommend that a dopamine agonist must be used before levodopa.

◆ Dopamine agonists can be used alone in monotherapy or in combinations with other medications.

◆ Dopamine agonists are longer-acting than levodopa.

◆ The most concerning side effect to monitor is impulse control disorder.

◆ Another concerning side effect is sudden sleepiness (which may affect driving).

Considerations for Dopamine Agonists

There was an early notion that use of dopamine agonists would delay the initial occurrence of motor fluctuations and dyskinesias. Clinical studies have shown that pramipexole, for example, may slightly delay the onset of motor fluctuations and dyskinesias; however, there was no difference in long-term motor symptoms and mortality. These studies also revealed that, compared to those receiving levodopa, people receiving dopamine agonists had an overall less robust improvement in their motor symptoms, a lesser quality of life, and a higher burden of non-motor side effects. The idea that dopamine agonists should be the first line of therapy has largely been debunked by multiple studies. Dopamine agonists or levodopa preparations can both be used as the first agent in the treatment of the Parkinson's disease motor symptoms. The choice should be individualized and made after a detailed discussion with a doctor. There are important differences between levodopa and dopamine agonists. For example, dopamine agonists (especially long-acting formulations) can be administered less frequently during the day than most levodopa preparations. This could be a major factor in deciding to use dopamine agonists before levodopa preparations.

Commonly, dopamine agonists are also utilized as an add-on treatment to levodopa in an effort to increase the duration and smoothness of the treatment effect. This approach has been recommended for relatively younger individuals with Parkinson's disease; however, the definition of younger is yet to be defined. Most experts agree that all of the dopamine agonists are roughly as effective in monotherapy or in combination with other drugs.

Monoamine Oxidase Type B Inhibitors (MAO-B Inhibitors)

Dopamine, when released into synapse (the communication channel) between brain cells, after binding with the dopamine receptor, detaches and is quickly reabsorbed into the brain cell from which it was released. Within the brain cell, dopamine is broken down by an enzyme called

IMPULSE CONTROL DISORDER

Impulse control disorder in Parkinson's disease is characterized by the development of a new or heightened obsession with an activity that previously was not important. These activities are usually rewarding, but in ICD the person does them to an extreme. Common examples include:

- Gambling
- Shopping
- Sex
- Eating

Note: Certain factors may increase the risk of ICD, including male gender, history of addiction, history of anxiety, history of anger, history of obsessive-compulsive traits, and younger age.

CASE EXAMPLE   AMANDA

Amanda is a 45-year-old woman who has been diagnosed with Parkinson's disease for the past four years. She visits the neurologist with her spouse. She has been doing very well on ropinirole (3mg, three times a day). Upon examination, her tremors, rigidity, and bradykinesia are well controlled. She denies any notable side effects, including sleepiness. Her spouse reports that Amanda has been shopping compulsively (even for items she does not need) and is painting many hours each day. She continues with these activities at the expense of her sleep, family activities, and financial well-being.

The neurologist explains that these are symptoms consistent with ICD and are associated with the use of ropinirole. Amanda has a long-standing history of obsessive-compulsive traits, and while this does not concern her, her family is very concerned.

The neurologist clarifies that these ICD symptoms need to be treated, because, if left unchecked, they can cause psychological distress, financial ruin, and relationship problems.

There is one option, the neurologist says: "Amanda needs to stop the use of ropinirole and use levodopa as a dopamine replacement." Amanda and her spouse ask the neurologist the following questions:

Can Amanda switch to another dopamine agonist, such as pramipexole or rotigotine?
No. This side effect is a class side effect of dopamine agonists, which means it can be caused with any of these medications. Replacing ropinirole with pramipexole will not decrease the ICD symptoms.

Can Amanda decrease the dose of ropinirole rather than stopping it?
Although decreasing the dose of ropinirole might cause an initial decrease in the ICD symptoms, the symptoms have a tendency to reappear. ICD symptoms can occur with any dose of dopamine agonists, but a higher dose can worsen them.

How should Amanda stop her ropinirole?
It is very important that Amanda slowly decreases the ropinirole. This applies to all dopamine agonists. A sudden stop can be associated with withdrawal symptoms. Even with a slow decline, Amanda needs to watch for withdrawal symptoms, which are referred to as "dopamine agonist withdrawal syndrome" (DAWS).

Amanda then begins taking carbidopa/levodopa (25/100mg at an initial dose of one tablet three times a day) in addition to ropinirole. She tolerates the addition of levodopa without issues. She decreases ropinirole and notices that she is nauseated, irritable, and has decreased motivation. She remembers that her doctor told her to expect a "rocky period" as she transitions from ropinirole to levodopa, so she decides to "power through" these symptoms.

When Amanda completely discontinues her ropinirole, she does not feel well. She is nauseated, anxious, depressed, occasionally confused, constantly tired, and dizzy when standing up. She contacts her neurologist for an urgent visit. The neurologist diagnoses her with DAWS.

Amanda is restarted on a small dose of ropinirole. When she reaches 0.5mg three times a day, she reports that she no longer has the symptoms of nausea, anxiety, and depression. She continues to take carbidopa/levodopa (with the dose adjusted for better motor symptom control). She continues to have ICD symptoms, which are monitored by her spouse and with the assistance of a mental health counselor.

monoamine oxidase type B (MAO-B). Parkinson's disease experts use drugs called "MAO-B inhibitors" at low dosages to block the breakdown of levodopa and increase the amount of dopamine available in the brain, which can be helpful for Parkinson's disease symptoms.

Some examples of MAO-B inhibitors approved for the treatment of Parkinson's disease are selegiline (pill and dissolvable form), rasagiline, and safinamide. Although selegiline and rasagiline can be used as monotherapy, overall, their effect(s) on the motor symptoms are much weaker than that of either levodopa or dopamine agonists. In addition to monotherapy, MAO-B inhibitors can be used as add-on therapy, usually added to dopamine agonists and/or levodopa. There has been some debate about the use of rasagiline to delay disease progression (i.e., as a neuroprotective), but there has been wide debate and the FDA panel that was convened to address this question ruled that rasagiline could not be labeled as a neuroprotective drug. The benefits of selegiline, rasagiline, and safinamide have not been tested head to head. Some experts prefer selegiline for treatment of symptoms such as walking issues (as it contains an amphetamine metabolite). Safinamide has not been shown effective as monotherapy but may be added to other Parkinson's disease drugs. Safinamide has yet to reveal any increased benefits.

MAO-B inhibitors are in general well-tolerated and there are few safety issues. Side effects may include headache, dizziness, insomnia, and nausea. At the recommended low dosages used for Parkinson's disease, the risk of drug-drug interaction and risks of mixing with antidepressants remains very low. Most Parkinson's disease experts routinely use low-dose MAO-B inhibitors and antidepressants together. Many doctors will also stop MAO-B inhibitors a week or more before surgery because of potential side effects with anaesthetics and pain medications.

THINGS TO KNOW ABOUT THE USE OF MAO-B INHIBITORS

◆ These drugs have only very small symptomatic effects and they cannot replace levodopa or dopamine agonists.

◆ These drugs can be used in monotherapy or in combination with other medications.

◆ To date there has not been overwhelming evidence that these drugs are neuroprotective.

◆ The risk of an adverse event from mixing a low-dose MAO-B with an antidepressant is very low because it would take high doses of the MAO-B to activate the MAO-A receptor and thus result in the side effects.

Catechol-O-Methyl Transferase (COMT) Inhibitors

Dopamine and levodopa can be broken down by an enzyme called catechol-O-methyl transferase (COMT). This enzyme is present not only in the brain, but also throughout the body. COMT inhibitors work by blocking this enzyme, thereby increasing the amount of dopamine and levodopa available to combat the symptoms of Parkinson's disease.

Entacapone is currently the most commonly used COMT inhibitor. It does not cross the blood-brain barrier and acts only on the COMT that is present outside of the brain.

Entacapone works by decreasing the amount of levodopa that is broken down before reaching the brain, and this improves Parkinson's disease symptoms. Entacapone is not recommended to be used on its own (monotherapy), as it must be used with levodopa to be effective. It is not recommended as an add-on treatment in early-stage Parkinson's disease, as studies have shown that it tends to increase the risk of motor fluctuations and dyskinesias. Entacapone is used for the management of motor fluctuations and to prevent the wearing off of Parkinson's disease medications between dosages, but, when used, it can worsen symptoms. Entacapone is usually well-tolerated, and the most common side effect is nausea. Other side effects may include stomach and gastrointestinal symptoms, as well as fatigue and dizziness. Diarrhea and also slight discoloration of the urine are common.

Tolcapone is another COMT inhibiting drug. It can cross the blood-brain barrier. Tolcapone works on the brain COMT enzyme, and this leads to an increase in the levels of dopamine (similar in effect to MAO-B inhibitors). The use of tolcapone has significantly decreased due to a risk of liver toxicity, and regular blood tests to monitor for toxicity are required when taking this medication. Opicapone is a new once-a-day drug in this class that was recently FDA-approved.

THINGS TO KNOW ABOUT THE USE OF COMT INHIBITORS

◆ These medications may extend the effects of a dose of levodopa and can be used between dosages.

◆ These medications must be taken with carbidopa.

◆ Frequently, the dose of levodopa and/or agonists must be reduced to avoid dyskinesia when taken with COMT inhibitors.

◆ Diarrhea and discolored urine are common side effects.

Other Parkinson's Disease Agents

In addition to dopamine replacement, other strategies have been used to treat the motor symptoms in Parkinson's disease. Amantadine, istradefylline, and multiple anticholinergic agents are examples of such strategies.

Amantadine

This is an anti-influenza medication that was decommissioned by the U.S. FDA. In the late 1960s, in a serendipitous discovery, neurologists at Harvard University noticed that Parkinson's disease patients given this medication for flu prophylaxis experienced improvements in symptoms. Amantadine can be used as monotherapy or as an add-on treatment. Its beneficial motor effects are much less than observed in levodopa preparations or in dopamine agonists. It is preferred by some providers in patients who have a predominance of tremors, although its best use has been dyskinesia suppression and the management of motor fluctuations. Possible side effects include swelling of the ankles and discoloration of the legs (both of these effects are usually mild, and in most cases not a cause to stop treatment). Amantadine may also contribute to or cause hallucinations, nightmares, and confusion.

Istradefylline

This is an adenosine A2A receptor antagonist. In addition to dopamine, other neurotransmitters are involved in Parkinson's disease, including glutamate and adenosine. Early-stage studies of istradefylline have shown that blocking the function of the adenosine A2A receptor can improve the symptoms of Parkinson's disease. In addition to istradefylline, there are multiple agents with similar mechanisms of action that are currently being developed. Istradefylline is not recommended as monotherapy. It is considered as an add-on treatment to levodopa and is now approved in the U.S. and Japan.

Anticholinergic Medications

Anticholinergic medications include agents such as trihexyphenidyl and benztropine. Anticholinergics are mainly used for the treatment of a tremor in Parkinson's disease, but in some cases they may improve other symptoms. This class of medication was developed in the 19th century for the management of Parkinson's disease, but they are now rarely used, due to their poor effect in controlling the symptoms of rigidity and bradykinesia (slowness), but also because of their side effects. The most notable side effects from anticholinergic therapy include confusion, hallucinations, vision changes, dryness in the mouth, skin rash, and constipation. These medications are usually reserved for younger and cognitively normal patients with Parkinson's disease, especially if tremors are a major and disabling symptom. Many experts do not use anticholinergics at all because of the risk of cognitive dysfunction. There is also emerging evidence that long-term use may be associated with dementia.

CASE EXAMPLE · HANK

Hank is a 58-year-old right-handed man with a history of high blood pressure. He seeks a neurologist for evaluation of the symptoms of rest tremor of the right hand that may be associated with clumsiness. He tells the doctor his symptoms began six months ago. The neurologist confirms the diagnosis of Parkinson's disease but is very sensitive when delivering the diagnosis. She emphasizes that this is not Alzheimer's disease, that this is very treatable, and that there is a path to a happy and productive life. She discusses with Hank how the symptoms will progress slowly over the years, and she explains the brain changes that may occur as a result of Parkinson's disease. She tells him that the current treatments improve the symptoms and quality of life, but that they may not change the progression of the disease.

Hank explains that he wants to start treatment, as the tremor and clumsiness are bothering him and disrupting his work. After a discussion about the different treatment options, Hank's preference is to start with carbidopa/levodopa (25/100mg taken as one tablet, three times a day). His choice is based on the fact that he works as a machinist and will require the best symptom control. He is aware of warnings on the internet not to take levodopa, but his doctor assures him of its safety and the risk/benefit ratio.

COMMONLY APPROVED MEDICATIONS

The following summaries of commonly approved Parkinson's disease medications and their dosages are provided courtesy of and with permission from the Parkinson's Foundation educational series on Parkinson's disease medications. More details on all of these medications can be found at Parkinson.org.

MEDICATIONS CURRENTLY APPROVED FOR TREATMENT OF PARKINSON'S DISEASE	
Class/Type	**Medication**
L-Dopa	Carbidopa/levodopa (Sinemet)
	Carbidopa/levodopa orally disintegrating tablet (Parcopa)
	Carbidopa/levodopa controlled release (Sinemet CR)
	Carbidopa/levodopa/entacapone (Stalevo)
	Carbidopa/levodopa extended release capsules (Rytary)
	Carbidopa/levodopa enteral suspension (Duopa)
	Note: This is a gel formulation of the drug that requires a surgically placed tube.
Dopamine agonists	Apomorphine (Apokyn)
	Bromocriptine (Parlodel)
	Pramipexole (Mirapex)
	Pramipexole dihydrochloride extended release (Mirapex ER)
	Ropinirole (Requip)
	Ropinirole extended-release tablets (Requip XLTM)
	Rotigotine transdermal system (Neupro)
COMT inhibitors	Entacapone (Comtan)
	Tolcapone (Tasmar)
MAO-B inhibitors	Rasagiline (Azilect)
	Selegiline or deprenyl (Eldepryl)
	Selegiline HCl orally disintegrating tablet (Zelapar)
	Safinamide (Xadago)
Anticholinergics	Benztropine mesylate (Cogentin)
	Procyclidine (not currently available in the U.S.)
	Trihexyphenidyl (Artane)
Other	Amantadine extended release (Gocovri)
	Droxidopa (Northera)
	Pimavanserin (Nuplazid)
	Rivastigmine tartrate (Exelon)

MEDICATION (PRODUCT NAME IN PARENTHESES)	DOSAGES IN MILLIGRAMS (TABLETS UNLESS OTHERWISE NOTED)	TYPICAL TREATMENT REGIMENS	POTENTIAL SIDE EFFECTS	INDICATIONS FOR USAGE (ITALICS = APPROVED BY U.S. FDA)
LEVODOPA				
Carbidopa/ levodopa immediate release (Sinemet)	10/100, 25/100, 25/250	150–1000mg of levodopa total daily dose (divided 3–4 times)	Low blood pressure, nausea, confusion, dyskinesia	*Monotherapy or combination therapy* for slowness, stiffness, and tremor
Carbidopa/ levodopa orally disintegrating (Parcopa)	10/100, 25/100, 25/250	150–1000mg of levodopa total daily dose (divided 3–4 times)	Same as above	Same as above, plus need for dissolvable medication in mouth, especially if swallowing is impaired
Carbidopa/ levodopa extended release (Sinemet CR)	25/100, 50/200	150–1000mg of levodopa in divided doses, depending on daily need	Same as above	*Monotherapy or combination therapy* for slowness, stiffness, and tremor
Carbidopa/ levodopa entacapone (Stalevo) [See COMT inhibitors below]	12.5/50/200, 18.75/75/200, 25/100/200, 31.25/125/200, 37.5/150/200, 50/200/200	150–1000mg of levodopa total daily dose, depending on daily need	Same as above, plus diarrhea and discolored urine (due to entacapone)	*Replacement for carbidopa/ levodopa* for motor fluctuations (benefit of entacapone)
Carbidopa/ levodopa extended-release capsules (Rytary)	23.75/95, 36.25/145, 48.75/195, 61.25/245	855–2340mg of levodopa total daily dose	Same as above	*Monotherapy or adjunct therapy* for slowness, stiffness, and tremor; Note: Dosages of Rytary are not interchangeable with other carbidopa/ levodopa products
Carbidopa/ levodopa enteral solution (Duopa)	Clinician-determined	Up to 2000mg of levodopa over 16 hours	Same as above	For the treatment of motor fluctuations in patients with advanced Parkinson's disease

MEDICATION (PRODUCT NAME IN PARENTHESES)	DOSAGES IN MILLIGRAMS (TABLETS UNLESS OTHERWISE NOTED)	TYPICAL TREATMENT REGIMENS	POTENTIAL SIDE EFFECTS	INDICATIONS FOR USAGE (ITALICS = APPROVED BY U.S. FDA)
DOPAMINE AGONISTS				
Ropinirole (Requip)	0.25, 0.5, 1, 2, 3, 4, 5	9–24mg total daily dose (divided 3–4 times)	Low blood pressure, nausea, leg swelling and discoloration, confusion, sleep attacks, compulsive behaviors	*Monotherapy or combination therapy* for slowness, stiffness, and tremor
Ropinirole XL (Requip XL)	2, 4, 6, 8, 12	8–24mg once per day	Same as above	Same as above
Pramipexole (Mirapex)	0.125, 0.25, 0.5, 0.75, 1, 1.5	1.5–4.5mg total daily dose (divided 3–4 times)	Same as above	Same as above
Pramipexole ER (Mirapex ER)	0.375, 0.75, 1.5, 2.25, 3, 3.75, 4.5	1.5–4.5mg once per day	Same as above	Same as above
Rotigotine (Neupro)	1, 2, 3, 4, 6, 8 patch	4–8mg once per day	Same as above	Same as above; patch delivery an advantage for some
Apomorphine (Apokyn)	30mg/3ml vial	2–6mg	Significant nausea; must take anti-nausea medication with dose, especially when starting therapy	*Adjunct therapy* for sudden wearing off; the only injectable, fast-acting dopaminergic drug
MAO-B INHIBITORS				
Selegiline (l-deprenyl, Eldepryl)	5	5mg once or twice per day	Nausea, dry mouth, light-headedness, constipation; may worsen dyskinesia; possible rare interaction with antidepressants and other drug classes	*Monotherapy* for slowness, stiffness, and tremor; *adjunct therapy* for motor fluctuations
Rasagiline (Azilect)	0.5, 1.0	1mg once per day	Same as above	Same as above

MEDICATION (PRODUCT NAME IN PARENTHESES)	DOSAGES IN MILLIGRAMS (TABLETS UNLESS OTHERWISE NOTED)	TYPICAL TREATMENT REGIMENS	POTENTIAL SIDE EFFECTS	INDICATIONS FOR USAGE (ITALICS = APPROVED BY U.S. FDA)
Selegiline HCL orally disintegrating (Zelapar)	1.25, 2.5	1.25–2.5mg once per day	Same as above	Same as above, plus need for dissolvable medication in mouth (absorbed in mouth)
COMT INHIBITORS				
Entacapone (Comtan)	200	200mg 4–8 times daily (with each levodopa dose)	Diarrhea, discolored urine, plus enhancing side effects of levodopa, especially dyskinesia and confusion	*Combination therapy with levodopa* for motor fluctuations (not pharmacologically active by itself)
Tolcapone (Tasmar)	100, 200	100mg up to 3 times daily	Same as above, plus increased risk of liver inflammation	Same as above (second-line due to side effects)
OTHER ANTI-PARKINSON'S MEDICATIONS				
Amantadine (Symmetrel)	100mg capsules; 50mg/5ml syrup	100mg 2–3 times daily	Nausea, confusion, leg discoloration (livedo reticularis), mild anticholinergic effects (see below)	*Monotherapy* for slowness, stiffness, and tremor; *combination therapy* with levodopa for levodopa-induced motor fluctuations; especially helpful for suppressing dyskinesia
ANTICHOLINERGICS				
Trihexyphenidyl (formerly Artane)	2, 5mg tablets; 2mg/5ml elixir	1–2mg 2–3 times daily	Confusion, memory issues, hallucinations, dry mouth, blurry vision, urinary retention	*Monotherapy or combination therapy,* predominantly for tremor in younger people; should be avoided in elderly
Benztropine (Cogentin)	0.5, 1, 2	0.5–2mg 2–3 times daily	Same as above	Same as above

Assessing the Most Bothersome Symptoms

Early in Parkinson's disease, changes in walking respond well to levodopa or dopamine agonists. These changes may be more related to stiffness and/or slowness of movements, and seem to be related to dopamine pathways in the brain. Later in Parkinson's disease, walking problems become less responsive to levodopa or dopamine agonists, as they seem to be related to dysfunction in non-dopamine pathways, and treatment is more difficult.

It is important to identify the most bothersome symptoms when deciding which medication to choose. In this chapter, we have focused our discussion on the treatment options for three motor symptoms: tremor, stiffness (rigidity), and slowness (bradykinesia). In addition, there are other motor symptoms that can affect individuals with Parkinson's disease, such as walking and balance problems, speech impairment, and swallowing difficulties. For a discussion of the treatment of non-motor symptoms in Parkinson's disease, such as memory changes, please consult Chapter 5.

Walking problems and similar motor symptoms do not usually respond well to the treatment options we have discussed thus far. Hence, if the patient with Parkinson's disease is not bothered by their tremors, but is significantly bothered by their balance issues, treatment with levodopa might not offer a significant reprieve. This seems to be related to the fact that, in addition to the dysfunction in the dopamine pathways, dysfunction in other neurotransmitter pathways occurs in Parkinson's disease, especially as the disease progresses. These include neurotransmitters such as glutamate, adrenaline, and acetylcholine. Studies involving medications that can increase the levels of acetylcholine (such as donepezil and rivastigmine), which are also medications used to treat dementia in Parkinson's disease (see Chapter 8), are not consistent in their findings. Some studies show a possible improvement in walking and others do not. Moreover, medications that can increase glutamate and adrenaline in the brain failed to cause an improvement in walking.

Physical therapy, occupational therapy, and speech therapy provide some benefits in the management of these other motor symptoms (see Chapter 2).

Disease Progression

As Parkinson's disease progresses and motor dopamine-producing cells are lost, treatment complications usually begin to slowly appear. These complications can be separated into two groups: motor fluctuations and dyskinesia.

Motor Fluctuations

After taking levodopa or dopamine agonist, a person will start feeling the positive effects on the tremors and stiffness (usually within 30 minutes). This positive effect on the motor symptoms is commonly referred to as the "ON" state. By contrast, the "OFF" state refers to the condition when the effect of the medications decreases, wears off, or stops. In the early stage of Parkinson's disease, patients will only feel the "ON" state as long as they stay on the medication schedule. This effect of medication in the early stage of Parkinson's disease has been referred to as the "honeymoon." As the disease progresses, the "ON" state lasts for shorter and shorter periods of time, and the "OFF" state becomes more noticeable. The occurrence of these fluctuating "ON" and "OFF" periods has been referred to as motor fluctuations.

COMMON MOTOR FLUCTUATIONS	EXAMPLE
Predictable "OFF"	Julie takes her pramipexole pills three times a day, five hours apart. She tells her doctor that the "ON" state lasts four hours and that, one hour prior to each dose, she feels that she is in the "OFF" state.
Unpredictable "OFF"	Sam takes carbidopa/levodopa five times a day, four hours apart. He tells his doctor that the duration of the "ON" state is not predictable, as it can vary from two to four hours.
Sudden "OFF"	Rhonda tells her doctor that she occasionally feels a sudden occurrence of an "OFF" state, as if all the dopamine has left her body at once. She feels very stiff and immobile.

Dyskinesia

This refers to the development of unwanted movements. The movements are a result of both disease progression and the use of medications related to dopamine. The unwanted movements can result in stiffening of a joint (dystonia) or excessive flowing or dance-like movements (chorea). The dyskinesia(s) can occur either in the "ON" state (peak-dose dyskinesia), "OFF" state (OFF dyskinesia), or during the transition between the "ON" and "OFF" states (biphasic or diphasic dyskinesia). The most common dyskinesias occur in the "ON" state as the dopamine reaches its highest level in the bloodstream. In this scenario, there are too many movements rather than too few, as is expected in Parkinson's disease.

The motor fluctuations and dyskinesia can have an impact on quality of life. They can also become frequent and, when prominent, many patients refer to them as "the roller coaster ride"—up when "ON" and down when "OFF."

INHALED LEVODOPA AND CARBIDOPA-LEVODOPA GEL

There is a new and recently available inhaled form of levodopa called Inbrija. This type of inhaled levodopa may be useful for sudden "OFF" periods or times when the dopamine levels become unexpectedly low. The trials of this medication included patients taking carbidopa/levodopa—this is important because the carbidopa in the bloodstream may be necessary to combat potential nausea.

Duopa is an intestinal gel formulation of carbidopa-levodopa that is delivered through a tube into the intestine. This therapy provides two main benefits: a reduction of "OFF" time and an increase in "ON" time without significant dyskinesia. These benefits may result from a more steady level of levodopa in the blood and/or from bypassing the stomach (which, in Parkinson's disease, can be sluggish, resulting in erratic absorption). Duopa requires evaluation by a multidisciplinary team including the neurologist, a specialized nurse, and the gastroenterology specialist, and also requires family support. Given the complexity of the Duopa procedure and the expertise needed for follow-up and adjustments, Duopa is limited to specialized centers and to patients who have adequate caregivers.

Management Options for Motor Fluctuations and Dyskinesias

There are multiple approaches to treating motor fluctuations and dyskinesia(s). The most important step in treatment of motor fluctuations and dyskinesia is to identify the type of the complication and to pin down when it occurs.

Management Options for Motor Fluctuations

1. Take medications more frequently—for example, if the "ON" effect lasts three hours, but the time between doses is four hours, then take the doses every three hours.
2. Supplement the carbidopa/levodopa treatment with other longer-acting medications (such as dopamine agonists or amantadine).
3. Switch to a longer-acting formulation (such as carbidopa/levodopa ER, pramipexole ER, rotigotine patch).
4. Add an MAO-I inhibitor or COMT inhibitor.
5. Use apomorphine injections or inhaled levodopa.
6. Consider advanced therapies, such as Duopa or deep brain stimulation (DBS).

Management Options for Dyskinesias

1. Decrease the dose of short-acting dopaminergic medications.
2. Supplement the carbidopa/levodopa treatment with other longer-acting medications (such as dopamine agonists).
3. Switch to a longer-acting formulation (such as carbidopa/levodopa ER, pramipexole ER, rotigotine patch).
4. Use amantadine or similar preparations.
5. Consider Duopa or DBS.

A Concluding Note: Participating in Clinical Trials

In this chapter, we have discussed treatment options available at the time of the writing of this book. These options are constantly changing and newer treatments may become available. Prior to release on the market, medications are tested in multiple stages: initially, in animal models and cell cultures, then, later, in humans.

It is through the selflessness of human volunteers that newer medications and novel approaches to treatment eventually become available. Dr. Okun's book *Parkinson's Treatment: 10 Secrets to a Happier Life* stresses that one of the most important tips is to ask what is new in Parkinson's disease research and treatment at every visit with the doctor.

As a participant in clinical trials, a person with Parkinson's disease has access to cutting-edge technologies and medication. Multiple university-affiliated and independent centers offer opportunities to participate in clinical trials. Patients with an interest in clinical trials can discuss this with their treating doctor. More information about the available studies can be found on the Clinical Trials website run by the U.S. National Library of Medicine (www.clinicaltrials.gov). This website lists the study site, the study steps and protocol, and contact information. Note, however, that this government-sponsored site does not offer any indication on the quality of the study, so it is important to read about the study and discuss the pros and cons with a doctor treating Parkinson's to obtain help in deciding which study to choose.

The Office for Human Research Protections (OHRS), part of the U.S. Department of Health and Human Services (HHS), has excellent resources about research studies, the volunteer's rights, and general information about study protocols. These resources can be accessed via the HHS (www.hhs.gov).

MEDICATION FOR PARKINSON'S DISEASE MOTOR SYMPTOMS

I believe in prescription drugs.
I believe in feeling better.
— DENIS LEARY

➤ Take the amount of medication you need to control your symptoms.

➤ If you are just changing the dose and not the time intervals in Parkinson's disease, you are probably doing something wrong.

➤ MAO-B inhibitors (selegiline, zydis selegiline, rasagiline, Xadago) provide very mild symptomatic effects and are not replacements for dopamine agonists or dopamine replacement.

➤ MAO-B inhibitors have not been definitively proven to be neuroprotective or to slow clinical disease progression.

➤ One in five to six people who start a dopamine agonist will develop an impulse control disorder. Always have a spouse or friend monitor for impulse control disorders when starting a dopamine agonist.

➤ Levodopa (Sinemet), especially at high dosages, can, rarely, result in manic behavior (hyperactive state) and compulsive sexual behavior, including possible strange behaviors.

➤ Dopamine extenders, such as entacapone and Stalevo, may require reduction in other dopamine dosages to lessen the risk of dyskinesia.

➤ The Duopa dopamine pump is a gel form of dopamine that can be continuously infused into the small intestine. The most common side effects from the pump are related to issues with the tube.

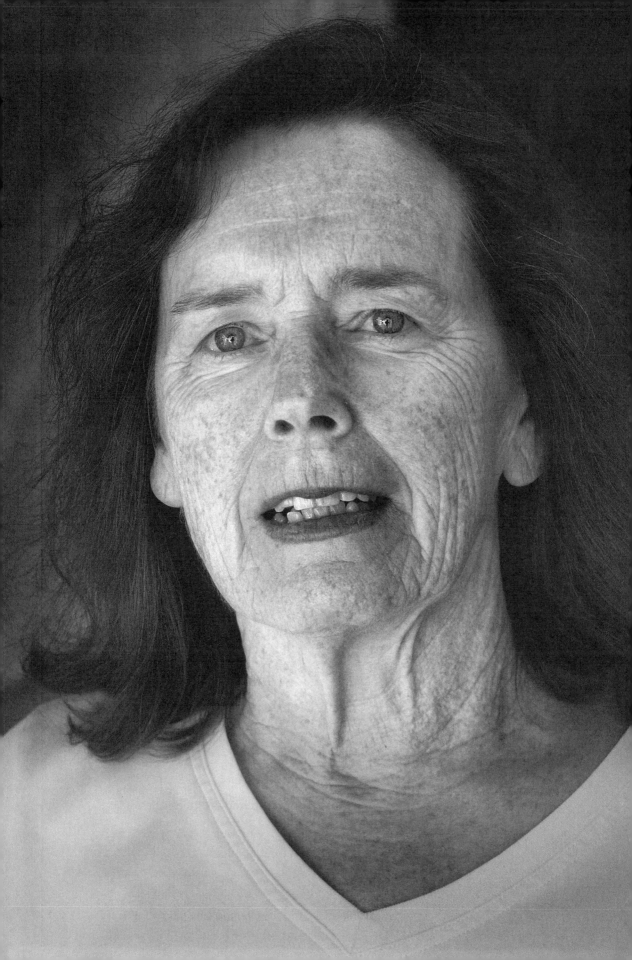

MEDICATIONS FOR NON-MOTOR PARKINSON'S DISEASE SYMPTOMS

Once you choose hope,
anything is possible.
– Christopher Reeve

MANAGING PARKINSON'S DISEASE is frequently a "head to toe and beyond" endeavor, and it is key not to miss the complexities of the disease, particularly those that are not easily visible. Many "invisible" symptoms—referred to as "non-motor" symptoms—can be effectively managed with the right strategies and medications. These strategies have been shown to improve quality of life. In this chapter, we will review the management strategies helpful for non-motor symptoms, including those affecting the gastrointestinal system, the genitourinary system, and the cardiovascular system, as well as quality of sleep. Discussion of mood and other non-motor symptoms related to cognition and thinking will be covered in Chapter 8.

Sialorrhea (Drooling)

Saliva is not produced more quickly in people with Parkinson's disease. However, over time, some Parkinson's disease patients do seem to swallow less frequently and less effectively than people without Parkinson's disease.

This leads to an imbalance of the normal production and clearance of saliva, which can lead to pooling of secretions and to drooling.

Treatment Options for Drooling

There are several habits and treatment options that can help address drooling in Parkinson's disease. Here are a few to consider.

Taking Frequent Sips of Water

This is a conservative option used to trigger swallowing. This is a particularly good strategy in a social setting.

Sucking on Candy or Chewing Gum

Both of these approaches can trigger swallowing.

Applying Atropine Eye Drops Under The Tongue

A 1-percent ophthalmic atropine solution can be administered, one to two drops at a time, three times a day. Very rarely, this could lead to a side effect of confusion or hallucinations.

Medications

All of the medications to decrease drooling have higher risks for systemic side effects, such as confusion, hallucinations, constipation, or blurred vision, and are usually avoided in Parkinson's disease patients. Medications in this category include "anticholinergics" such as glycopyrrolate (usually given as 1–2mg pills, two to three times daily, as needed) and scopolamine (1mg patch every two to three days; this is the same patch used for sea sickness). Other medications, such as trihexyphenidyl or diphenhydramine, are usually avoided because of hallucinations (trihexyphenidyl) and cognitive side effects.

Botulinum Toxin Injections

These injections in the salivary glands can be used to reduce the amount of saliva produced. This procedure usually involves a series of simple outpatient injections once every three to four months. The injections are administered to the lower cheek area and to an area just below the jawline. An experienced botulinum toxin injector can usually avoid the rare side effects, such as weakness of neighboring muscles (including facial muscles or swallowing muscles). Studies have shown that both botulinum toxin A and B seem to be effective against drooling.

→ **CLINICAL PEARL**

Botulinum toxin is typically injected into the parotid glands and submandibular glands (both salivary glands) to reduce drooling. Among brands of botulinum toxin, only incobotulinumtoxinA (Xeomin) is approved for sialorrhea, at a dose of 100 units injected once every 16 weeks (30 units into each parotid gland and 20 units into each submandibular gland). Botulinum toxin B has recently been FDA-approved and should be used at 1500-3500 units intraglandularly divided in four injection sites. Typically the clinician injects 500-1500 units in the parotid gland and 250 units in submandibular gland on each side of the face.

Constipation

One of the most universal and earliest symptoms of Parkinson's disease is constipation. It can be debilitating. In many cases it is a "premotor symptom" that offers an early clue to the diagnosis of Parkinson's disease. Parkinson's disease patients frequently complain of a reduction in the number and/or frequency of stools, hard stools, bloating, and abdominal cramping.

Gastroparesis

This is when the stomach is not able to properly empty its contents and can result in bloating, discomfort, and early satiety (feeling full). The changes in gastrointestinal movement can be important, as they may affect how consistently a person is able to absorb his or her medication. When severe constipation occurs, a gastric emptying study, or gastric scintigraphy, may be performed to assess the severity of delay in intestinal movements. In some cases, prescription medication is required to stimulate movement.

Useful Strategies to Treat Constipation

There are several methods and habits that can help address constipation in Parkinson's disease. Here are a few strategies to consider.

Water

An easy, inexpensive, and highly effective approach: drink more water! The gastrointestinal tract and the intestines need water to move and eventually expel stool. Traditionally, six to eight glasses (8oz each) of fluid per day has been recommended, excluding carbonated and caffeinated beverages.

Fiber

Natural sources of fiber that can supplement the diet include fruits and vegetables, cereals, and snacks. Over-the-counter supplements can be helpful, but these supplements require water to be effective. The supplements often pull water into the gut, so if you are not drinking, they can potentially lead to dehydration.

Probiotics

These substances are over-the-counter, and while there are

few studies, they are safe and many patients report that they are useful.

Activity

Exercise promotes bowel health and inactivity worsens constipation. Going for a walk or exercising on a recumbent bike can be helpful for constipation.

Position

The "squatting position" when defecating has been considered conducive and natural for helping bowel movements. Placing a footstool under your feet can help to achieve an optimal position to address constipation.

Medications

Lubiprostone revealed a benefit for patients with Parkinson's disease enrolled in a clinical trial. Over-the-counter options can work to increase the bulk of stool and draw in fluid to facilitate movement, or they can stimulate a bowel movement. There are also multiple routes of administration of medications and some routes may be preferred over others as a personal preference.

GASTRIC EMPTYING STUDY

In this kind of study, a person ingests food with a radioactive tracer in it and pictures are taken of the gut at multiple points in time to determine how much dye is retained in the stomach as compared to a normal condition. When gastric (stomach) emptying time is too long, the Parkinson's disease pills may not be absorbing. It is important to have treatment of this condition to avoid serious and rare complications such as intestinal obstruction.

Laxatives

Some laxatives can affect electrolyte balance (such as magnesium, calcium, and sodium). The effects of electrolyte imbalance should not be underestimated. There can be resultant heart rhythm changes or other health complications. Some laxatives may also result in cramping or gas, or even drug dependence. It is important to talk to a doctor about all health conditions and medications to avoid unexpected risks of laxatives or drug-drug interactions.

Mechanisms of Action for Laxatives

There are many different types of laxatives, with different ways of acting upon the body. Here are a few to consider.

Bulk Producing

These laxatives provide a substance that, when taken with water, can promote a bulkier and softer stool that is easier to pass. Examples include psyllium husk powder (such as Metamucil), methylcellulose (Citrucel), guar gum (Benefiber), and calcium polycarbophil (such as FiberCon). Water consumption is critically important to support the mechanism of action of laxatives. Bulk producing laxatives may produce results in one to three days.

Osmotic Laxatives

These laxatives increase the flow of water into the colon and facilitate stool passage. Examples include magnesium hydroxide (Milk of Magnesia), polyethylene glycol (MiraLax), lactulose, and sorbitol. Some osmotic laxatives contain sugar molecules, which may be an important consideration for diabetics. Results from osmotic laxatives commonly occur in one to three days.

Stool Softeners (Emollient Laxatives)

These laxatives contain surfactants, which help wet the stool and prepare it for easier passage. An example includes

---

→ CLINICAL PEARL

Metoclopramide (Reglan) is a medication used to treat gastroparesis. But a caution: It is absolutely not recommended in Parkinson's disease! It can cause worsening of symptoms of Parkinson's disease and cause dystonia (involuntary muscle contraction that can cause twisting or pulling) and other movement disorders.

docuate (Colace). These may take a week or more to
take effect.

Bowel Stimulants

These work by triggering intestinal contractions to move
stool through the colon. Examples include bisacodyl
(Correctol, Dulcolax), senna derivatives (Senokot), and castor
oil. Effects can be quick, but cramping and diarrhea may
occur. Prolonged use is not recommended because of the
risk of dependence.

Suppositories

Suppositories are medications that are inserted into the
rectum (about one inch), past the anal sphincter. These
medications stimulate contractions that help expel stool.
Typically, these are bullet-shaped and may contain stimulant
laxatives or lubricants. Examples include biscodyl (Dulcolax)
and glycerin (Fleet, Pedia-Lax).

Enemas

This is a process of injecting fluid into the rectum by
inserting a tube that allows the fluid to flow into the colon.
This type of laxative procedure may be necessary when stool
is impacted, but is not recommended for routine use. Enemas
may contain mineral oil, sodium phosphate, or bisacodyl.

PRACTICAL TIP

Be sure to ask your doctor or pharmacist to review your medications and
supplements for any medications that can cause constipation. These include:

- Opioids and pain pills
- Amantadine
- Iron supplements
- Anticholinergic medications
- Some blood pressure medications

Urinary Issues

Dysautonomia, or dysfunction of the "autopilot" system of the body, can occur in Parkinson's disease. Many functions that are automatically regulated may slip into a state of imbalance. In Parkinson's disease, overactive bladder (also referred to as neurogenic detrusor overactivity) is more common than underactivity. This overactivity can result in a frequent urgency to urinate, an increase in the frequency of nighttime urination, and, in some cases, incontinence. An overactive bladder, coupled with problems with mobility, will present difficulties for a Parkinson's disease patient trying to get to the bathroom quickly.

Some Medications Used to Treat Urinary Issues

Here are a few common medications that might be considered for urinary issues in Parkinson's disease.

Anticholinergics

These medications can help in reducing overactive involuntary bladder contraction. However, anticholinergics can result in confusion, thinking problems, hallucinations, or worsening constipation. The risk of these side effects increases with age.

Mirabegron

This medication has a novel mechanism of action: it stimulates "beta-3 adrenergic" receptors. Mirabegron improves urinary urgency and incontinence in Parkinson's disease patients and may be another option to consider, especially if side effects occur with anticholinergic medications.

Desmopressin

This medication mimics the effects of a natural hormone called "anti-diuretic hormone" or ADH. Desmopressin was tried in a 1995 study (published in *Movement Disorders*) with a small number of Parkinson's disease patients and was shown to help five of eight patients with nighttime frequent urination. However, three of eight patients had to stop taking the medication due to the side effects of confusion and low sodium. We do not use this medication in our practice.

Amantadine

This is a medication used to treat dyskinesia and other symptoms of Parkinson's disease that has also been reported to decrease urinary frequency, urgency, and incontinence.

More About Anticholinergics

A recent study of solifenacin (Vesicare) was conducted in 23 Parkinson's disease patients. Solifenacin is an anticholinergic with a more selective profile in the exact types of receptors it blocks in the brain, which may have fewer cognitive effects. There was a reduction in the number of episodes of urination per day, a reduction in the number of nighttime urinations, and a reduction in incontinence episodes. The benefit of this drug has to be weighed against the risk of side effects, as it is still an anticholinergic and, therefore, may affect cognition. Side effects can include dry mouth, dizziness, headaches, and, especially, cognitive issues.

Other anticholinergics, such as diphenhydramine (Benadryl) and trihexyphenidyl (Artane), have been used in Parkinson's disease, but their use has been severely limited due to the common occurrence of cognitive issues. Oxybutynin, trospium chloride, and tolterodine are anticholinergics used for overactive bladder. Tolterodine

---

MEDICATIONS TO TREAT PARKINSON'S DISEASE URINARY SYMPTOMS

- Anticholinergics, such as solifenacin (Vesicare)— but watch for side effects (especially cognitive)

- Mirabegron, which is a beta-3 adrenergic

- Desmopressin (high-risk drug)

- Amantadine

has been shown in recent studies to be associated with a significant reduction of overactive bladder symptoms; however, constipation and dizziness or headache were common side effects.

Non-Pill-Based Approaches to Urinary Symptoms

There are also a number of ways to address urinary issues that do not involve medications. Here are a few to consider.

Botulinum Toxin

This can be injected into the bladder wall in an effort to control an overactive bladder. It works primarily by reducing the amount of the chemical neurotransmitter acetylcholine. This chemical is released from the nerve endings, but blocking it by botulinum toxin results in relaxation of the bladder. The advantage of using this localized approach is that it does not affect the brain, and thus cognitive side effects do not occur. The approach requires a specialist, typically a urologist, who must pass a scope through the urethra. The urologist then passes a small needle through the scope and makes several focused injections into the bladder. This treatment has been shown to reduce urinary frequency and incontinence; however, there is some risk, making it somewhat impractical. Chronic treatment requires a procedure every three to four months. This approach may also not be optimal in patients prone to urinary tract infections.

Electrical Stimulation of the Tibial Nerve in the Lower Leg

This approach, called "percutaneous nerve stimulation" (PTNS), has been rarely used to address urinary symptoms. The therapy sends impulses backward, up to the bladder, in order to inhibit the reflex nerve pathways, which can ultimately stimulate bladder contractions. This therapy has been shown to reduce overactive bladder symptoms, including urinary frequency and incontinence, in some Parkinson's disease patients. The therapy was tested in a small group of patients over 12 sessions and there were no serious side effects.

Sacral Nerve Stimulation (Neuromodulation)

This is another approach that uses an implanted device to stimulate the sacral nerve. The device can be controlled by an external remote and the delivery of stimulation is aimed at reducing bladder contractions. Implantation requires a surgical procedure. Usually, prior to the implantation of a long-term device, a test trial can be performed. The lead, or wire, is placed where the sacral nerve emerges, at a location in the lower back called the "sacral foramen." Imaging is used to guide the wire placement and the wire is threaded into the buttock area. A permanent battery can be implanted if stimulation using the temporary one is helpful. Sacral nerve stimulation has been shown to reduce urinary frequency and urgency in some people with bladder issues, though there has not been extensive research in Parkinson's disease.

Fluid Intake

Drinking fluids liberally early in the day but reducing the intake of fluids after dinner can help reduce the nocturnal need to urinate, but it can also contribute to dehydration. For some people, wearing protective briefs or pads can help reduce the stress of incontinence accidents overnight or when traveling outside of the home. A urinal at the bedside can be used to prevent falling in the middle of the night, especially if multiple trips per night to the bathroom are needed.

Pelvic Rehabilitation Therapy

This specialized form of physical therapy involves learning and practicing exercises to strengthen the pelvic floor muscles. Small, early studies suggest that pelvic floor muscle exercises and bladder training utilize biofeedback with muscle sensors (electromyography, or EMG sensors, placed on muscles record feedback that can be visualized on a television screen). This approach may reduce nighttime urination, urinary incontinence, and symptoms of overactive bladder. This type of therapy may not be available in all cities.

Physical and Occupational Therapy

Physical and occupational therapists can be helpful in developing a plan to optimize safety, especially for overnight trips to the bathroom. Some examples include advising on best care strategies, such as grab bars, illumination of the walking path (such as a night light), or other strategies to avoid falls (e.g., bedside urinals).

Erectile Dysfunction (ED)

Sexual health has a tremendous impact on quality of life. In Parkinson's disease, the management of erectile dysfunction (ED) is handled in fundamentally the same manner as in the general population. Medical conditions that can result in or contribute to ED should be addressed. The safety of potential medication trials should be assessed. Sildenafil (Viagra) was studied in a small number (20) of Parkinson's disease patients and was shown to be effective. This medication and others in the same class of phosphodiesterase type 5 (PDE5) inhibitors can carry the risk of worsening orthostatic hypotension (dizziness and low blood pressure), especially in Parkinson's disease. The potential benefit has to be weighed against risk. Other medications used for this problem, including tadalafil (Cialis), may be tried as well, although there is less published in Parkinson's disease on this medication. Sildenafil lasts four to six hours and tadalafil lasts up to 18 hours.

There may also be individual differences in cost and insurance coverage.

Orthostatic Hypotension (OH)

Orthostatic hypotension, which is a sudden drop in blood pressure after changes in position (sitting, standing, lying), is important to diagnose and to address. Orthostatic hypotension carries a risk of syncope (passing out), falling, and injury. Dizziness or falls commonly occur almost immediately after standing. Many emergency room and general doctors will spend a lot of time and money attending to Parkinson's disease patients for the many causes of syncope. The most common cause of syncope in Parkinson's disease is orthostatic hypotension.

The first step in managing orthostatic hypotension involves increasing hydration. In order for blood to circulate to the brain, there has to be adequate volume within the blood vessels, and this comes from being well hydrated. Imagine watering a garden with a hose turned partially on or with a hose that has very little water available—this would limit the ability to get water to its intended destination. In addition to the typical, traditional advice of drinking six to eight 8oz glasses of water per day, it is important to be sure that medications being taken are not affecting hydration levels, as is the case with a diuretic or a water pill. Finally, many autonomic nervous system experts believe that drinking a tall, cold glass of water in the morning is a good treatment for orthostasis.

DAILY ACTIVITIES THAT CAN HELP MANAGE ORTHOSTATIC HYPOTENSION

◆ Drink two large (cold) glasses of water in the morning to start the day.

◆ Sit on the edge of the bed for a few seconds or minutes before standing.

◆ Pump the legs before standing, or bring your knees to your chest a few times in bed before getting up.

Strategies for Managing Orthostatic Hypotension

Here are a few common strategies that may be used to address orthostatic hypotension in Parkinson's disease.

Compression Stockings

These function as a mechanical aid to facilitate circulation by increasing the (venous) return of blood flow. For optimal effect, these need to be worn high on the leg.

Abdominal Binders

These may provide an alternative to compression stockings, which can be difficult for individuals with Parkinson's disease to put on and take off.

Liberal Use of Salt

If safe from a medical standpoint, increasing salt intake can be helpful because salt pulls fluid into the blood vessels, increasing volume and enhancing circulation (one of the few reasons that a doctor may recommend eating more salt!).

MORE TIPS FOR MANAGING ORTHOSTATIC HYPOTENSION

- Avoid certain common medications that can aggravate or cause orthostatic hypotension, including bladder, pain, and prostate medications.

- Hydrate (drink lots of water).

- Do active exercises before getting up from bed.

- Use mechanical aids, such as compression stockings or abdominal binders.

- Discuss medications with your doctor, such as fludrocortisone, midodrine, droxidopa, pyridostigmine, or possibly atomoxetine.

- Watch for supine hypertension as a side effect.

The remaining medication strategies are generally aimed at either increasing fluid or increasing the tone of blood vessels. Fludrocortisone is a medicine that is called a "mineralocorticoid"—a medication that works by pulling fluid into the blood vessels. Another orthostatic hypotension medication is midodrine, which is an "alpha-adrenergic" agonist that works by stimulating the sympathetic nerve receptors located directly on blood vessels. A newer drug, droxidopa, works similarly to increase the sympathetic tone in blood vessels, but its mechanism of action is different: it is converted to norepinephrine, and that stimulates the receptors to improve orthostatic hypotension. Finally, an older drug, pyridostigmine, works to slow the breakdown and increase the availability of a chemical called acetylcholine, which is a neurotransmitter that facilitates messaging between nerves as well as between nerves and muscle. The messaging can sometimes be improved by this medication and result in improvements of orthostatic hypotension. Pyridostigmine seems to be the least effective of the treatment measures.

Cautions When Using Orthostatic Hypotension Drugs

Side effects of orthostatic hypotension strategies are important to consider when choosing a medication. Fludrocortisone can result in sodium retention and supine hypertension, meaning that it can increase the blood pressure when lying down. For this reason, fludrocortisone is usually taken early in the day and not before naps or bedtime. Fludrocortisone use can also lead to low potassium and to ankle swelling. The risks of higher blood pressure and of electrolyte changes have to be considered, especially in patients with preexisting heart and kidney problems. Midodrine, like fludrocortisone, can also cause supine hypertension and should not be taken before lying down. Midodrine may cause or aggravate urinary retention. As urinary issues are already common in Parkinson's disease, the risk must be balanced when selecting a particular medication. Droxidopa and midodrine both carry black box warnings for the risk of supine hypertension. A 2018 study published in *Movement Disorders* showed that the impact of droxidopa may be reduced by taking high doses of carbidopa, though the exact threshold for that effect was not clear. Pyridostigmine has a more modest effect on orthostatic hypotension and may cause an increase in salivary secretions and diarrhea (but supine hypertension is not a concern).

Supine hypertension may be a consequence of medications, but it can also be neurogenic, which means it can happen in 50 percent of Parkinson's disease patients. Tilting the bed 30 to 45 degrees to elevate the head may be helpful. Very rarely, a short-acting anti-hypertensive (blood pressure reducing pill) may be required; however, we try to avoid this approach if possible.

These are only the most common side effects—the exhaustive list of possible side effects for all of these medications is much longer. Norepinephrine transporter inhibitors are a less commonly used class of medications for orthostatic hypotension and include the attention deficit hyperactivity disorder (ADHD) medication atomoxetine. These medications have the potential to increase the availability of the chemical norepinephrine. Sometimes this approach can inadvertently stimulate the brain's norepinephrine receptors and may lead to side effects such as weight loss, nausea, insomnia, and severe hepatitis.

CASE EXAMPLE HELEN

Helen is a 78-year-old woman with Parkinson's disease. She has been falling frequently. After talking through the circumstances of her falls, it becomes apparent that most occur moments after standing, or in the morning as she gets out of bed. Sometimes she feels light-headed getting out of a chair or standing from squatting. This seems worse when she gardens in the sun.

Her medications include carbidopa/levodopa (25/100, two pills every four hours between eight o'clock in the morning and midnight) and pramipexole (1.5mg three times daily), which she has taken for at least five years.

In the clinic, Helen's blood pressure in the seated position is 132/83. After standing for three minutes, her blood pressure drops to 83/55. Her doctor determines that she is experiencing orthostatic hypotension.

Helen's doctor advises her to increase her fluid intake and to use salt more liberally in her diet. This leads to some improvement in the frequency and severity of her symptoms. The next step is for her to wean off pramipexole and to slightly increase her carbidopa/levodopa. Although she had tolerated that medication for a long time, with age, her body composition and her Parkinson's disease needs changed, and this medication is no longer the best option.

Helen's doctor also reviews medications for orthostatic hypotension with her, and a plan is made to add a medication if the first round of changes does not provide enough relief. The therapeutic goal is not to maintain an ideal blood pressure at all times, which is not always possible, but to minimize the symptoms of the blood pressure drops, including falls, dizziness, or transient confusion.

In some severe cases, where very high and very low blood pressures occur, more complicated treatment plans may be needed to more closely adjust medication according to blood pressure readings.

Combination therapy to treat orthostatic hypotension is often necessary. Even with combinations of medications, the problem can be difficult to manage. Some people may be susceptible to orthostatic hypotension and it may be triggered by eating a large meal, as the blood vessels of the gut dilate to aid digestion. The dilation of the blood vessels may divert blood from the brain to other organs. Eating smaller, more frequent meals can help avoid this complication. Some sufferers of orthostatic hypotension find that caffeine with a meal can be helpful.

In summary, multiple strategies are available to treat orthostatic hypotension. Fine-tuning behavioral and medication approaches is the best management strategy. It is important to remember that the most accurate measurement of blood pressure is approximately 60 to 90 minutes after taking dopamine medication, because dopamine replacement therapies typically reduce blood pressure.

Sleep Disorders

Tiredness and sleep difficulty are common in Parkinson's disease. Parkinson's disease affects the brainstem and hypothalamus by depositing abnormal proteins and also by disrupting the circuitry in the areas of the brain contributing to sleep-wake cycles (also referred to as the "circadian system"). Dopamine has a major role in influencing the human circadian system, and the deficiency of dopamine in Parkinson's disease likely has a direct impact on sleep and wake balance. There are also many other chemicals and areas of the brain, besides the dopamine system, that are implicated in Parkinson's disease and the sleep-wake system. When approaching sleep issues in a Parkinson's disease patient, we suggest uncovering the daytime and nighttime behaviors surrounding wakefulness and sleep, and asking the

> **DID YOU KNOW?**
>
> Sleep dysfunction occurs in up to 98 percent of people with Parkinson's disease. It is an important non-motor symptom to address.

bed partner about behaviors during sleep. The underlying reasons for poor sleep dictate the optimal intervention, and one very important aspect to a complete assessment is to undergo a sleep study.

Strategies to Improve Sleep in Parkinson's Disease

It is very important to address sleep issues in Parkinson's disease. Here are a few strategies that can help improve sleep.

Minimize Daytime Sleepiness

Many medications may compound fatigue, which is a common symptom of Parkinson's disease. It is important for people with Parkinson's disease to review medications with their pharmacist and care team to be sure that any unnecessary medications that may contribute to daytime sleepiness can be minimized. Daytime napping and excessive tiredness during the day are red flags that there may be a sleep disorder. Short naps can be a restorative strategy, especially when a brief "power nap" facilitates a recharge in energy level. Prolonged naps can lead to resetting of the sleep clock and to impairment in the ability to rest, especially later in the night. Napping can, in some cases, lead to a vicious cycle of poor sleep, daytime tiredness, and a need to nap again. Although many medications exacerbate sleepiness, some medications stimulate wakefulness and result in insomnia—one example is selegiline when utilized late in the day.

→ **CLINICAL PEARL**

Optimizing Parkinson's disease medications may help with sleep. Trials involving levodopa and several dopamine agonists have shown that sleep improved, along with motor control.

TIPS FOR GOOD SLEEP HYGIENE

◆ Dim the lights one hour before bedtime.

◆ Avoid stimulating activity one hour before bedtime.

◆ Have a quiet, comfortable bedroom (this includes temperature setting).

◆ Use the bed only for sleep or sex.

◆ Avoid caffeine after lunch.

◆ Avoid bright screens at bedtime (if you read off of a screen, be sure to change the setting to the dimmest backlight).

◆ Limit daytime naps to 30 minutes.

◆ Do aerobic exercise during the day to improve sleep quality at night (a little bit goes a long way; avoid exercise right before bedtime).

◆ If you are awake for a prolonged period during the night, get out of bed and try going back to bed again when sleepy.

◆ Maintain a regular sleep schedule.

MORE TIPS TO ADDRESS SLEEP ISSUES

◆ Adjust the dose and timing of medications.

◆ Consider slow-release formulations of dopaminergics at bedtime or an optional overnight dose.

◆ Re-dose when waking at night.

◆ Add a medication such as a benzodiazepine (e.g., clonazepam), melatonin, or a cannabinoid.

Improve Sleep Hygiene

Sleep hygiene refers to the habits utilized to potentially improve or to worsen sleep. A tip for sleep hygiene is to reduce or dim light an hour or so before bedtime. Light stimulates the brain to suppress a chemical called melatonin. Melatonin provides the internal signal for sleep at night. Electronic devices, such as phones, computers, and electronic book readers, suppress melatonin and delay sleep onset. If these devices are used before bedtime, it is recommended to reduce the background lighting or to choose a night setting. Stimulating activities, such as physical exercise or stressful activities, are best shifted to earlier in the day, to facilitate a "winding down" period before bedtime.

Reduce Anxiety

Anxiety can also be a cause of delayed sleep onset. Racing thoughts, stress, and excessive worry can be clues to suggest that anxiety is taking effect. Some people with Parkinson's disease have generalized anxiety or anxiety when their dopaminergic medication wears off. When appropriate, treatment of anxiety may improve sleep (see Chapter 8). Some anxiolytic medications may be intentionally selected for their sedating properties and preferentially used at night. Similarly, untreated depression or psychosis can also interfere with sleep and, when clinically disruptive, need to be addressed. Untreated mood disorders can also lead to early-morning awakenings.

Other Sleep Considerations with Parkinson's Disease

There are a few more sleep-related issues that may arise in Parkinson's disease. Here are some further considerations.

Timing of Motor Symptom Medications

Too much or too little of these medications can have an impact on sleep.

Dyskinesia (Excessive Movement)

This is often caused by too much dopaminergic medication and may affect sleep. Reducing dopaminergic medication dosages at bedtime may be useful.

Erratic Medication Absorption

Erratic medication absorption can result from changes in gut motility or the microbiome, leading to erratic "ON" and "OFF" periods (as described in Chapter 4). This may potentially have an impact on sleep.

Wearing Off of Medicine

This can lead to disruption of sleep and spontaneous arousals. This has also been referred to as "reemergence of Parkinson's symptoms" and sometimes requires re-dosing dopaminergics. Cramps of the legs or toe curling, along with stiff and slow movement, are signs of this problem.

Drenching Sweats

This may occur from wearing off of dopaminergics in the middle of the night and may require longer-acting medications or re-dosing dopaminergics.

FUN FACT

Since the laws have been rapidly changing, many patients have been using cannabinoids and CBD oils to improve sleep. There are very few studies to support the use of cannabinoids and CBD oils in Parkinson's disease. If you use a cannabinoid or CBD oil for sleep, check with your doctor and set up a monitoring program to evaluate dose, response, and side effects.

Restless Legs Syndrome (RLS)

RLS is a condition that occurs when a person tries to rest quietly, especially at night, but is overcome by a restless and uncomfortable feeling. This feeling is so uncomfortable that it becomes necessary to move to relieve the inner sensation of discomfort. The feeling can be a painful, crampy, or tingly ("creepy crawly"), and can result in other indistinct but bothersome characteristics. Although the legs are most commonly affected, other body parts can be involved, especially over time. Usually, the problem occurs at night, but may occur after prolonged sitting.

RLS can sometimes be a sign of iron deficiency. A marker of iron deficiency is a low ferritin level and, if this is detected, iron replacement may improve the RLS symptoms. Constipation may be a side effect of iron supplementation, so water and fiber are important if treatment is pursued. Treatment of iron deficiency may not, in some cases, improve the RLS. Some medications and dietary triggers can contribute to RLS, such as antidepressants, caffeine, or red wine.

In Parkinson's disease, RLS may be a signal that dopaminergic medication is wearing off. In these cases, adjusting timing of medication or adding a long-acting medication at bedtime may help. Often, RLS may be present despite the lack of obvious modifiable triggers. In these cases, medications may be necessary. Treatment involves optimizing the Parkinson's disease medication regimen. One potential challenge is that many patients may already be on dopaminergics.

Medication Options for RLS

Here are some of the medication treatment options for restless leg syndrome in Parkinson's disease.

Dopamine Agonist Medications

These include pramipexole and ropinirole, which are available in short- and long-acting forms. Rotigotine, a patch with a 24-hour delivery system, is one available dopamine agonist. Possible side effects include tiredness, sleep attacks (sudden unwanted sleep), dizziness, nausea, swelling, and compulsive or impulsive behavior. Typical doses used for RLS treatment are pramipexole (0.125–0.5mg at night), ropinirole (0.25–4mg at night) or ropinirole (1–3mg patch applied daily). For those already taking a dopamine agonist, this may not be an effective approach for Parkinson's disease RLS.

Medications That Enhance "GABA"

Medications that enhance the brain chemical GABA can be efficacious in managing RLS. GABA is an inhibitory or blocking type of chemical in the brain. These medications include gabapentin and pregabalin in shorter- and longer-acting forms. Only gabapentin enacarbil is FDA-approved for moderate to severe RLS (600mg at night), though the other formulations are commonly used. Gabapentin (100–600mg at night) and pregabalin (150–450mg daily) are prescribed for RLS, though doses need to be reduced for elderly patients or for those with kidney trouble. The important side effects can include tiredness, confusion, cloudy thinking, worsening balance, falls, and weight gain. Some of these adverse events (tiredness, cognitive, and balance trouble) may overlap with the symptoms of Parkinson's disease and may thus make them worse. Therefore, these medications should be used with caution and at the lowest effective dose.

Levodopa

Immediate release or longer-acting levodopa may help RLS. If the last doses of the day are too early, wearing off overnight can lead to RLS. Sometimes, taking a slower-release levodopa at bedtime can help avoid overnight loss of benefit. Other times, taking a dose as needed when woken up in the middle of the night by symptoms can be an effective strategy. Side effects are consistent with other applications of levodopa (see Chapter 4). Note that if levodopa is already optimized, this may not be an effective treatment for Parkinson's disease–related RLS.

Benzodiazepines

Medications like clonazepam can alleviate RLS and also potentially treat REM behavioral disorder if present (see the following section). The risks include cognitive side effects, impaired balance, falls, and sleepiness. There has been an increased awareness and focus on risk to cognition, because patients on these medications report having a higher risk of impaired cognition. Examining the impaired cognition can be difficult, however, as many conditions that impair cognition have been associated with sleep disorders requiring the use of these medications, so the risks and benefits must be carefully weighed with a medical team. There is also mild concern that this class of medications may be habit-forming for a select group of people, so it is important to adhere closely to the prescribed instructions.

COMMON SLEEP DISORDERS

Other sleep disorders are also common in Parkinson's disease. Sleep apnea is one example and it is more common in Parkinson's disease than in the general population. Individuals with sleep apnea may experience snoring and a period where breathing appears to be interrupted. In the untreated state, it causes micro-arousals, meaning that the sleep pattern is disrupted without the person being consciously aware there is an issue. Daytime sleepiness and falling asleep unintentionally are common symptoms and, if not addressed, risk of high blood pressure and cardiovascular events (including stroke) is increased. Treatment commonly involves wearing a device, such as a mask, which provides positive airway pressure. Following treatment of sleep apnea, many Parkinson's disease patients report less daytime sleepiness and decreased fatigue. A sleep study is necessary for diagnosis of sleep apnea.

WHAT IS "AUGMENTATION"?

Augmentation is the worsening of RLS symptoms, potentially involving more body regions, occurring earlier in the day or following increasingly brief periods of time sitting down. Dopamine agonists and levodopa may relieve symptoms but may also carry a risk for augmentation. If augmentation occurs, the doctor will need to change the treatment strategy.

REM Sleep Behavior Disorder (RBD)

There is a stage of sleep when the eyes move rapidly and people begin to dream. In rapid eye movement (REM) sleep, or deep dreaming sleep, all of the muscles should be immobile or paralyzed. This means that if a person is dreaming, for example, of fighting a predator or dribbling a basketball, they are still lying quietly in bed. Many people with Parkinson's disease, however, lose this "atonia," or paralysis, and will physically act out their dreams. This physical acting out can lead to flailing, punching, kicking, or rolling out of bed. There may also be verbalization and the content of the dreams may be threatening or scary. Often, this symptom is detected by bed partners, who are woken by the activity and movements.

The significance for the person with REM sleep behavioral disorder is a risk of injury (such as falling out of bed) and a risk of fragmented, non-restorative sleep. Safety precautions include bed rails or placing soft materials on the floor next to the bed. Some medications, such as antidepressants, may occasionally aggravate REM sleep behavioral disorder. A sleep study is useful for diagnosis. Not all cases of REM sleep behavioral disorder require treatment, but if there is significant risk of injury to the patient or bed partner or significant disruption in sleep, treatment should be pursued.

Medications for RBD

Here are some of the medication treatment options for REM sleep behavior disorder in Parkinson's disease.

Clonazepam

This benzodiazepine medication is commonly used for REM sleep behavioral disorder (at doses of 0.25–1mg taken before bed). Clonazepam is long-acting and has been shown in studies to reduce threatening dreams, movements, and injuries. This medication, however, can worsen obstructive sleep apnea and has a risk of cognitive side effects (confusion) and exacerbating balance problems. Other benzodiazepines, such as lorazepam and diazepam, are less commonly used, as they are shorter-acting. If the benzodiazepine leads to early-morning drowsiness, one practical tip is to give the medication earlier in the night (e.g., after or with dinner). Sometimes dose reduction, such as reducing to half a pill, can help as well.

Melatonin

Melatonin is a hormone secreted by a region in the brain called the pineal gland, which helps regulate the 24-hour circadian sleep-wake cycle. When light decreases, usually at night, melatonin secretion increases and signals to the body that it is time to sleep. Melatonin pills have been used to shift sleep cycles and for changes in time zones (jet lag). There is some evidence that melatonin improves REM sleep behavioral disorder, though it has not been studied in Parkinson's disease specifically. Doses that are reported to be effective are in the 3–12mg range, with an average dose of approximately 6mg. This dose is taken at bedtime, or ideally in advance of bedtime, and may improve stillness and acting out dreams.

Rivastigmine Patch

A small 2012 pilot study published in *Movement Disorders* examined the rivastigmine patch—which has traditionally been used as a memory medication (cholinesterase inhibitor)—in 12 patients with Parkinson's disease.

In this very small study, bed partners of Parkinson's patients reported less acting out of dreams. Interestingly, memory medicines (cholinesterase inhibitors) have also been reported to worsen REM sleep behavioral disorder, so the research is not conclusive.

A Concluding Note

Non-motor symptoms in Parkinson's disease have the potential to have major impacts on daily life and overall well-being. Recognizing and treating non-motor symptoms will improve quality of life in Parkinson's disease. In many cases, treatment of non-motor symptoms has a greater impact than treating the tremor, stiffness, or slowness common in Parkinson's disease.

MEDICATIONS FOR NON-MOTOR PARKINSON'S DISEASE SYMPTOMS

Worry never robs tomorrow of its sorrow,
it only saps today of its joy.
— LEO BUSCAGLIA

- The non-motor symptoms are more disabling than the motor symptoms of Parkinson's disease (tremor, stiffness, slowness).

- Do not be embarrassed to take an antidepressant.

- Do not hesitate to identify and treat anxiety.

- Determine whether anxiety occurs when wearing off medications and consider changes in medication timing.

- Treatment of non-motor symptoms will in many cases improve motor symptoms.

- Apathy is more common than depression in Parkinson's disease.

- Dopamine agonists and counseling therapy could be helpful for apathy.

- Support from a licensed clinical social worker or counseling therapist has been shown to enhance the effects of medication.

- Treat constipation aggressively, as it has a huge impact on quality of life.

- Pain medications are a common offender for causing constipation.

SELECTED REFERENCES

Chinnapongse R, Gullo K, Nemeth P, Zhang Y, Griggs L. Safety and efficacy of botulinum toxin type B for treatment of sialorrhea in Parkinson's disease: a prospective double-blind trial. *Movement Disorders*, 2012 Feb;27(2):219–26.

Di Giacopo R, Fasano A, Quaranta D, Della Marca G, Bove F, Bentivoglio AR. Rivastigmine as alternative treatment for refractory REM behavior disorder in Parkinson's disease. *Movement Disorders*, 2012 Apr;27(4):559–61.

Hajebrahimi S, Chapple CR, Pashazadeh F, Salehi-Pourmehr H. Management of neurogenic bladder in patients with Parkinson's disease: a systematic review. *Neurourology and Urodynamics*, 2019 Jan;38(1):31–62.

Li SX, Lam SP, Zhang J, et al. A prospective, naturalistic follow-up study of treatment outcomes with clonazepam in rapid eye movement sleep behavior disorder. *Sleep Medicine*, 2016;21:114–20.

Narayanaswami P, Geisbush T, Tarulli A, Raynor E, Gautam S, Tarsy D, Gronseth G. Drooling in Parkinson's disease: a randomized controlled trial of incobotulinum toxin A and meta-analysis of Botulinum toxins. *Parkinsonism & Related Disorders*, 2016 Sep;30:73–77.

Palleschi G, Pastore AL, Stocchi F, et al. Correlation between the overactive bladder questionnaire (OAB-q) and urodynamic data of Parkinson disease patients affected by neurogenic detrusor overactivity during antimuscarinic treatment. *Clinical Neuropharmacology*, 2006;29(4):220–29.

Palma JA, Kaufmann H. Treatment of autonomic dysfunction in Parkinson disease and other synucleinopathies. *Movement Disorders*, 2018 Mar;33(3):372–90.

St Louis EK, Boeve AR, Boeve BF. REM sleep behavior disorder in Parkinson's disease and other synucleinopathies. *Movement Disorders*, 2017 May;32(5):645–58.

Suchowersky O, Furtado S, Rohs G. Beneficial effect of intranasal desmopressin for nocturnal polyuria in Parkinson's disease. *Movement Disorders*, 1995;10:337–40.

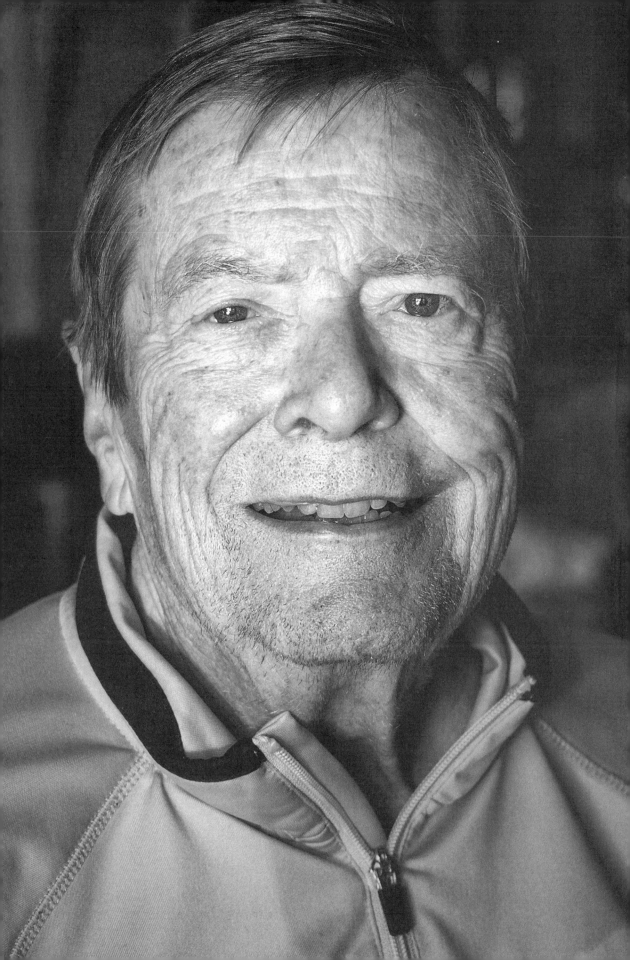

CHAPTER 6

SURGICAL THERAPIES FOR PARKINSON'S DISEASE

You have brains in your head.
You have feet in your shoes.
You can steer yourself in
any direction you choose.
– Dr. Seuss

THE NOTION THAT Parkinson's disease could be treated either by destroying brain tissue (e.g., ablative therapy) or by passing electrical current through it (e.g., deep brain stimulation) may seem outrageous, but advances in medicine have changed our reality. In this chapter, we will review and summarize what is known about each of the surgical approaches utilized for Parkinson's disease, and provide practical tips for patients who are considering an operation. Surgery for Parkinson's disease is not for everyone, but for a subset of patients, it can be life-changing.

The History of Parkinson's Disease Surgery

Surgical approaches to treating Parkinson's disease predated medication therapy, as levodopa (dopamine replacement) was not introduced until the late 1960s. During the many decades that patients were eagerly awaiting medical therapies for their Parkinson's disease symptoms, surgical approaches filled the void. Early innovators in the field observed patients with shaking and dance-like movements, called "chorea." Surgeons reasoned that they could simply cut the motor pathway in the brain and the shaking would cease. Unfortunately, although this approach helped with the movement, it also resulted in weakness. The trade-off was unacceptable: tremor for stroke relief.

Gradually, neurosurgeons began to migrate toward an approach that targeted a group of structures in the brain called the "basal ganglia." The exact function of the basal ganglia was unknown at the time, and surgeons, as well as leading neuroscientists, reasoned that these brain structures served as some sort of movement integrator. A well-known breakthrough came when Irving Cooper, a famous neurosurgeon at St. Barnabas Hospital in New York, tied off an artery called the "anterior choroidal" artery. The patient had Parkinson's disease and suffered from a debilitating tremor, but she was being operated on by her neurosurgeon for another reason. By tying off the anterior choroidal artery, Cooper inadvertently cut the blood supply to an area located in the basal ganglia called the "globus pallidus." The result was a stroke. The tremor stopped, but this time there was no accompanying weakness. Impressed by the outcome, Cooper began to purposely place lesions in the globus pallidus, either by injecting alcohol or by burning the tissue with a heated probe. He noticed that if he made the lesions too small, they would have no effect, and if he made them too big, he risked accidentally damaging the motor or visual pathways, leading to a stroke. Over the ensuing decades, neurosurgeons have improved the technique and now can target brain areas that correspond to specific Parkinson's disease symptoms.

Multidisciplinary Screening

The most critical step for the success of deep brain stimulation (DBS) surgery is comprehensive multidisciplinary screening. Many DBS centers pay lip service to this step and, when asked, they will usually answer, "Of course we have a multidisciplinary team." It is important for patients and families to be able to identify quality versus shabby DBS screening.

The first step in multidisciplinary screening is to consult a neurologist with expertise in movement disorders. A

COMMON BRAIN REGIONS TARGETED BY LESION (ABLATIVE) THERAPY

◆ Globus pallidus internus (GPi) lesion — The procedure is referred to as a "pallidotomy," and most lesions in this area improve tremor, stiffness, slowness, dyskinesia, and the smoothness of medication responses (enhancement of the Parkinson's disease "ON" state).

◆ Subthalamic nucleus (STN) lesion — The procedure is referred to as a "subthalamotomy" and, similar to pallidotomy, most lesions in this area improve tremor, stiffness, slowness, dyskinesia, and the smoothness of medication responses. Lesions of the subthalamic nucleus can occasionally result in hemiballismus, which is a wild, flinging movement.

◆ Ventralis intermedius nucleus of the thalamus (VIM) lesion — The procedure is referred to as a "thalamotomy," and most lesions in this brain area improve resting tremor.

◆ Lesion of the zona incerta or posterior subthalamic area — This has been used by some surgeons to target tremor or other Parkinson's disease symptoms.

neurologist who has completed fellowship training in Parkinson's disease and movement disorders would be ideal. The Parkinson's disease medications should be optimized with trials that include changes in dose, administration interval, and make-up of the cocktail of medications. The neurologist should discuss the details of the symptoms that may or may not improve following DBS therapy. Finally, the neurologist should perform a levodopa challenge test and record a scale, called the Unified Parkinson's Disease Rating Scale, both on and off dopaminergic medications (off medications for approximately 12 hours). The response to medications remains the single best predictor of DBS outcome. Response to medications is not the only outcome, however, and in some cases, tremor and dyskinesia will respond to DBS, even if resistant to medication.

Once a neurologist has optimized medication, performed an on/off dopaminergic medication challenge, and deemed the patient a potential candidate for surgery, it is time for the rest of the multidisciplinary team to become involved. One of the most important members of this team is the neuropsychologist. It is critical for patients and families to understand the difference between a neuropsychologist and a counseling psychologist. A neuropsychologist tests thinking and cognitive functions. A counseling psychologist offers therapy. An experienced neuropsychologist is the appropriate professional to participate in a DBS screening.

CHOOSING THE APPROACH TO DBS SURGERY

◆ **Option 1:** Unilateral — One DBS lead is placed on one side of the brain. As part of a predetermined plan, the second DBS lead, on the other side, is not placed or is deferred until symptoms on the other side of the body become troublesome enough to address.

◆ **Option 2:** Simultaneous/bilateral — Two DBS leads (one on each brain side) are placed in the same operation.

◆ **Option 3:** Staged — One lead is placed, and then, several weeks later, a second DBS lead is placed in the other side of the brain.

A battery of neuropsychological tests should be performed to determine if there are any issues, including the examination of multiple areas of thinking, beyond just memory testing. A neuropsychologist can perform brief screenings of mood (depression, anxiety, impulsivity, and other issues), but if available, a psychiatrist should be included as part of the team. For those without access to a psychiatrist in their community, it will be important for the neurologist and neuropsychologist to assess for any active psychiatric issues, hallucinations, paranoia, impulsivity, and/ or suicidality. All of these issues need to be addressed, and any other existing conditions (e.g., bipolar depression) need to be stabilized. One big advantage to going in person to see a psychiatrist for screening and later follow-up is that the majority of patients will have significant issues and will require ongoing treatment. Many studies have revealed that neuropsychological and psychiatric issues can have a major impact on the DBS outcome.

The neurosurgeon plays a pivotal role in screening for potential DBS candidates. The neurosurgeon will assess the diagnosis but also weigh other conditions, such as heart disease, chronic obstructive pulmonary disease (COPD), and hypertension. He or she needs to assess surgical risk, including whether there are any blood thinners or high-risk conditions. Untreated hypertension, for example, increases the risk of bleeding in DBS brain surgery. The surgeon will make recommendations on the appropriate brain target, whether to implant unilaterally or bilaterally, and whether to stage the operation.

"Staging" an operation is performed to reduce the risk of post-surgical adverse events. Staging the procedure is considered a safer approach, when it is possible.

Additional Specialists in a Multidisciplinary Team

There are a number of other specialists who are useful to employ in multidisciplinary screening (although not all centers will have access to these individuals). What follows is a description of many of these roles.

Physical Therapists

Physical therapists will evaluate walking, balance, and falling, and assess pre- and post-operative needs for assistive devices.

Occupational Therapists

These professionals are critical in assessing and improving the ability to perform activities necessary for daily living and in assessing symptoms on both sides of the body. They are also needed in order to make recommendations on unilateral versus bilateral surgery (one lead or two leads).

Speech and Swallowing Therapists

These therapists will evaluate the risks and benefits of a surgical intervention and assess the risk on worsening speech or swallowing, as well as the risk for aspiration pneumonia.

Social Workers

A social worker will facilitate important discussions about who will care for the patient pre- and post-operatively (including logistical issues, such as determining who will drive the patient to and from the hospital), and discuss any financial issues or burdens.

Nutritionists

These professionals will address issues related to body weight and nutrition, particularly in patients who have been rapidly losing weight or who have a low baseline body weight (less than 100 lbs), to decrease general surgical risk.

MEMBERS OF A DBS MULTIDISCIPLINARY TEAM

- Neurologist
- Neurosurgeon
- Neuropsychologist
- Psychiatrist
- Physical therapist
- Occupational therapist
- Speech and swallowing therapist
- Social worker
- Nutritionist

An Inter-Professional Approach

Each of the rehabilitation specialists may also recommend safety measures before or after the operation. For example, in some cases, a patient may be admitted for rehabilitation prior to the operation. This procedure is referred to as "prehabilitation." In another circumstance, an individual with swallowing difficulties may be operated on but not allowed to eat until a post-operative swallowing assessment is completed.

Once all of the members of a DBS multidisciplinary team meet, the next step is for everyone to sit in the same room and discuss all aspects of an individual case. Our team runs like the Supreme Court, where all justices speak once before any justice speaks twice. Also, we purposely plan the meeting so that the neurosurgeon speaks last. We do this to be sure that all opinions are considered before a final recommendation is constructed. The highest level of health care a patient can hope for, we say, is when people are talking behind his or her back. The multidisciplinary DBS process is designed to gather information and to arrive at a recommendation based on discussion among a group of experts. This inter-professional approach is, in our opinion, how all health care should be delivered.

PARKINSON'S DISEASE SYMPTOMS ADDRESSED BY DBS THERAPY

- Tremor
- Dyskinesia
- On-off fluctuations
- Off time
- Rigidity
- Bradykinesia

PARKINSON'S SYMPTOMS NOT ADDRESSED BY DBS THERAPY

- Gait
- Balance
- Speech
- Swallowing
- Cognition (thinking)

In some cases, walking and freezing will improve when in the best dopaminergic medication "ON" state

---

The last part of the process is a discussion with the Parkinson's disease patient and family. We share the risks and benefits and discuss recommendations. The final decision for or against surgery should remain with the patient and the family.

One important lesson we have learned about DBS screening is that the multidisciplinary team will play a critical role in identifying the symptoms an individual expects to improve following a DBS surgery. We have learned that if each member of the multidisciplinary team individually has a discussion with the patient considering surgery, expectations can be set and, in some cases, reset. One reason that DBS can be seen to fail is because it fails to meet expectations, the most common of which is a patient who expects walking and balance to improve post-DBS surgery.

DBS MULTIDISCIPLINARY SCREENING QUESTIONS

You should be prepared to answer the following questions during the DBS multidisciplinary screening:

◆ Can you list, in order, the symptoms that are most disabling to you?

◆ What Parkinson's disease symptoms must get better to make it worth undergoing brain surgery?

The "Fast Track" Process

Parkinson's disease DBS at the University of Florida has evolved and improved using a process called "fast track." Once an expert neurologist or movement-disorders neurologist has evaluated and optimized medications and other therapies in the Parkinson's disease patient, a two-day evaluation is set up for the patient to meet with all of the specialists. After all evaluations are completed, the specialists meet in person as a team. What follows is a summary of how the process operates. Versions of this process have been modified across the world based on resources and on expertise. In many cases, Parkinson's

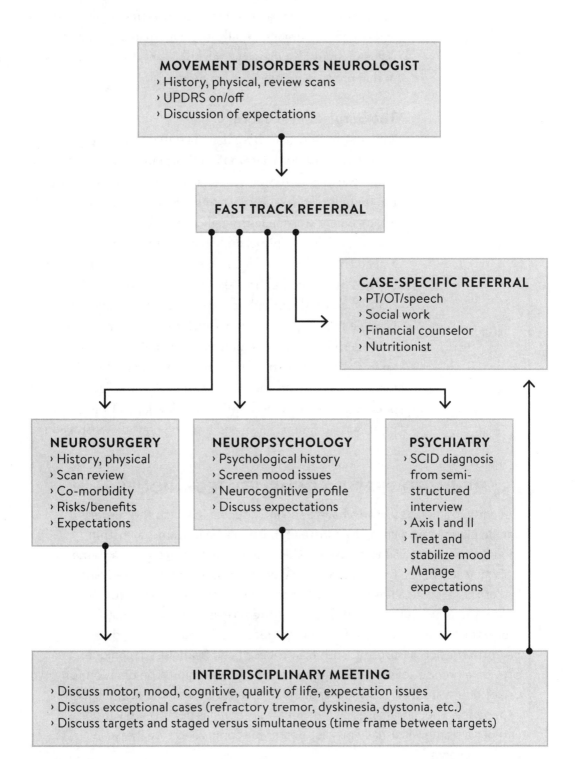

MOVEMENT DISORDERS NEUROLOGIST
› History, physical, review scans
› UPDRS on/off
› Discussion of expectations

FAST TRACK REFERRAL

CASE-SPECIFIC REFERRAL
› PT/OT/speech
› Social work
› Financial counselor
› Nutritionist

NEUROSURGERY
› History, physical
› Scan review
› Co-morbidity
› Risks/benefits
› Expectations

NEUROPSYCHOLOGY
› Psychological history
› Screen mood issues
› Neurocognitive profile
› Discuss expectations

PSYCHIATRY
› SCID diagnosis from semi-structured interview
› Axis I and II
› Treat and stabilize mood
› Manage expectations

INTERDISCIPLINARY MEETING
› Discuss motor, mood, cognitive, quality of life, expectation issues
› Discuss exceptional cases (refractory tremor, dyskinesia, dystonia, etc.)
› Discuss targets and staged versus simultaneous (time frame between targets)

Example of "fast track" multidisciplinary DBS evaluation

disease patients are encouraged to consider surgery. In other cases, there is a need for further testing or alternative approaches to surgery. Finally, there are patients who, following multidisciplinary evaluation, are deemed high-risk or inappropriate candidates for surgery.

The Surgical Procedure

The past two decades have demonstrated that, whether considering surgery that would involve either an ablative brain lesion or a DBS device, it is critical to precisely locate the brain target. In the 1950s and 1960s, an important advancement was made through the work of two German scientists (Ernest Spiegel and Henry Wycis), who developed a head frame that provided a reference for every point in the brain. This created a three-dimensional set of coordinates that, when used with atlases of brain anatomy, made it possible to navigate within millimeters of any brain target.

Modern technology combines this headframe system with an improved brain atlas and can even further refine the targeting and, ultimately, the accuracy of the surgery. Instead of depending on paper brain atlases developed from a few post-mortem brains, advanced imaging now allows surgeons

FRAME-BASED VERSUS FRAMELESS TECHNIQUES

Recently, frameless systems have been introduced, in which the surgery can be planned on a computer. Instead of using a head frame, a custom mount can be screwed to the skull, which some patients prefer to a frame (this may also be a bit speedier on the day of the surgery). The disadvantage is that there is a small risk for skin infection because the timeline for the procedure is extended: one day to place the screws and another day (or more) for the creation of the computer-generated mount required to perform the actual surgery. Both frame-based and frameless techniques provide a precise solution to target a specific brain region. The decision for use of one system versus another should be based on an individual surgeon's experience. The more cases an individual surgeon has performed with or without a frame will usually predict better outcomes and a decrease in adverse events.

to visualize and point to a specific brain target and to plan the surgery. The procedure has transformed from an all-day endeavor to one that requires just a few short hours.

The team decides on a frame-based versus a frameless approach. After this, they may have the option to use a tool called a "microelectrode" to refine the target. Another powerful technique is to use a high-quality MRI to superimpose a brain atlas and to add the information from the microelectrode mapping. Together, this information can provide a three-dimensional estimate on the location of a target the size of a peanut.

Once the mapping has been completed (or deferred), a neurosurgeon can either place a lesion probe in the brain and heat it up (thalamotomy, pallidotomy, subthalamotomy) or, alternatively, place a deep brain stimulator. This is an important part of the procedure because it marks the last chance to adjust the position of the lesion or the DBS lead. The surgeon can put a test probe or the actual DBS lead in place, and a neurologist or a physiologist can pass electricity through the brain. If the location is appropriate, the benefits and side effects are usually easily demonstrated. If an anticipated benefit is absent or an unintended side effect manifests, the location can be adjusted.

DURING SURGERY: AWAKE OR ASLEEP?

Many patients and families ask about DBS when awake versus asleep. The advantage to a procedure while asleep is mainly comfort for the patient. The advantage of a procedure while awake is that the patient can participate in the microelectrode recording and test stimulation process, which can enhance the outcome. We prefer, when possible, to perform the procedure while the patient is awake. It is also possible to perform a hybrid surgery for the small subset of patients who are anxious about being awake during the procedure: They can be put to sleep for most of the procedure and awakened briefly for testing. Procedures while patients are asleep can be offered in both frame and frameless approaches.

Once the lesion or DBS is placed, another important aspect of care is obtaining a post-operative image. This can either be a CT scan fused back to an MRI or, alternatively, an MRI scan. The DBS lead has four or eight small metal contacts on it and each will need to be activated by a procedure called a "monopolar threshold review." The benefits and side effects can be documented at each contact and at each voltage level. This information, in combination with the image, can help a team judge whether the DBS lead is appropriately placed.

Battery Placement

Following the placement of a DBS lead (or leads) into the brain, a second surgical procedure must be performed to connect the DBS system to a power source. The power source is a battery, a pacemaker, a neurostimulator, or an impulse generator (IPG). The surgeon must tunnel under the skin, forming a cavity stretching from the scalp to below the clavicle (or collarbone). This is the most common pacemaker placement, but, in some cases, it can be located in the abdomen. An interesting observation is that many patients complain more of the pain and discomfort from pacemaker placement than from the actual brain surgery.

During the multidisciplinary screening, it should be decided whether to use a conventional battery or a rechargeable device. Many patients will opt for a conventional (non-rechargeable) battery, which may last three to five years, rather than dealing with recharging weekly or every few days. The skin incision over the battery is the most common place for an infection to begin, and we teach patients to report any redness to the DBS team immediately.

Following DBS and pacemaker placement, programming by a neurologist, nurse, or other health-care provider can begin. A team often waits a month after the brain leads have been placed, to allow swelling to resolve. There may be a temporary "honeymoon effect" from any swelling, where symptoms resolve even though the device has not been activated. There are thousands of possible programming settings, and an experienced team will require several appointments over a period of three to six months to optimize the device. These appointments are necessary not only for optimization of the DBS device, but also for medication management, rehabilitation therapies, and monitoring for emergence of neuropsychiatric symptoms. Newer devices also provide programs that a patient can set on their own and report positive and/or negative effects to the clinician. Programs are ideal device management for patients who travel long distances. Once a final DBS setting has been chosen, in most cases, there will be little long-term deviation from the setting.

A DBS THERAPY MYTH

Many patients misunderstand DBS therapy, thinking that a simple tweak in programming will resolve symptoms that emerge later, such as walking, talking, and thinking problems. This is a myth. Also, as the pacemaker battery runs out, symptoms may reemerge, and therefore it is important to monitor and predict battery longevity at each programming visit.

Choosing the Best Brain Target

It is important for patients and families to appreciate that DBS is a process and that, as part of a process, there should be a discussion about the most appropriate target for an individual patient: subthalamic nucleus (STN) or globus pallidus interna (GPi). In our earlier published work (2005), we called into question the state of the field at the time, in which most DBS surgery used STN as a target, even though randomized studies had yet to be published. It was our view that the GPi target could become recognized as effective. Research findings in the field today (several randomized studies have been published) reveal that the STN and GPi targets have effects on motor symptoms that are roughly equivalent. We have continued to contribute to research that has changed the conventional thinking about DBS therapy for Parkinson's disease from a one-size-fits-all approach (STN as the default target) to choosing STN or GPi based on individual symptoms. Thus, the field has shifted to a precision medicine mindset.

ADVANTAGES OF STN DBS

◆ Decrease in medication required

◆ Less frequent battery changes

◆ More economical

ADVANTAGES OF GPI DBS

◆ Suppression of dyskinesia (involuntary movements)

◆ Easy programming

◆ Better flexibility in long-term medication management

STN VERSUS GPI

Our match ends in a draw—a particular DBS target should be chosen based on an individual patient's symptoms and needs.

Unilateral Versus Bilateral DBS

Parkinson's disease is by definition an asymmetric illness, meaning that it affects one side of the body more than the other. The only long-term data we have available is drawn from the unilateral NIH COMPARE trial, where 21 (48 percent) of the 44 patients in our cohort did not undergo bilateral implantation and were treated for an average of 3.5 years. Fourteen (67 percent) of patients had a GPi target. The most common reason for adding a second-sided DBS in our series was the inadequacy of single-sided DBS to address motor symptoms. Patient satisfaction with motor outcomes was the most common reason for not undergoing a second DBS surgery.

Those who chose a second DBS procedure had significantly more Parkinson's disease symptoms in general. Parkinson's disease patients who have the predominance of symptoms on one side seem to do well with a single DBS implantation. Also, the odds of proceeding to bilateral DBS was more than five times greater for STN than for GPi, meaning that those with low scores for Parkinson's disease symptoms and highly asymmetrical symptoms may be adequately treated in many cases by a single GPi DBS lead.

Unfortunately, this study is the only one available in the literature and we would benefit from a larger dataset.

Early Versus Earlier DBS

There has been quite a bit of confusion over the term "early DBS." Many clinicians and patients have interpreted this to mean intervention with a DBS device soon after the diagnosis of Parkinson's disease, but there is no evidence that early DBS is safe or prudent. In 2013, an important paper was published in the *New England Journal of Medicine* on neurostimulation for Parkinson's disease with early motor complications. It is important for patients and families to understand that this paper examined "earlier DBS" and not "early DBS." German and French centers undertook research with a group of patients whose average age was 52 and whose average disease duration was seven years. The patients randomized into two groups: those who had "earlier DBS" (motor fluctuations within the preceding two years) and those who received medical therapy. The "earlier DBS" patients experienced a better improvement in quality of life. The interpretation of this study is important for patients and families. For those with young-onset Parkinson's disease, it may be beneficial to undergo DBS therapy before motor fluctuations set in and worsen. This does not apply, however, to the majority of Parkinson's disease patients whose symptoms first appear in their 60s and 70s.

There is only one safety study published on "early DBS." In this study, 28 patients had bilateral STN DBS surgery before the onset of motor fluctuations. The authors showed that this approach was safe, but the study was not designed to detect a difference in clinical progression of the disease or other potential advantages. Therefore, based on the available data, we do not recommend "early" DBS at this time.

The Risks of DBS

It is important to remember that DBS is an elective procedure. We tell patients that, while the risks are small, if there is a side effect, it can be significant. The multidisciplinary DBS screening procedure has been able

An important consideration for patients and families is that placing a second DBS lead on the opposite side of the brain has been associated with a worsening in symptoms, including walking, balance, talking, and thinking.

to predict unintended hospitalization and worse quality-of-life outcomes. These findings are important, because if the health team identifies risk factors during the screening process, the presence of these factors may increase the chances for an adverse event later. If, for example, the screening process uncovers a cognitive problem, there may be a high risk of post-operative confusion and/or memory loss.

The most worrisome complications of DBS include infection, bleeding, and stroke. The implanted device does not have a blood supply, so if bacteria latches on to the lead or the neurostimulator battery, even the strongest antibiotic will not solve the problem. Most cases of infection start as an innocent redness in the skin around the incision, and, if not quickly cleared by antibiotics, the device(s) may need to be temporarily removed. In rare cases, infection can lead to abscess (a pocket of bacteria and puss) and sepsis (response to an infection that releases chemicals into the bloodstream) and can be life-threatening. Infection rates even in expert centers can be 5 percent or greater.

The other worrisome complication is bleeding and coincident stroke. Stroke is a circumstance where the brain tissue may be deprived of oxygen and die. The dead tissue results in stroke symptoms such as weakness, numbness, speech problems, swallowing problems, vision difficulties, and problems with walking and balance. Controlling blood pressure before and during surgery can decrease the occurrence of bleeding and strokes. Particularly useful is an MRI scan with contrast, which is administered through an IV and outlines the blood vessels, so the neurosurgeon can choose a path for the DBS lead that will avoid bleeding. The overall occurrence of bleeding and stroke in well-selected patients is usually less than 5 percent.

Age should also be discussed when considering the risks and benefits of DBS. In general (but not in all cases), older age increases the risks of complications following DBS surgery, and many neurosurgeons become more cautious in patients over the age of 70 or 75. It is important to assess the physical frailty of each patient, as well as atrophy (brain shrinkage). Excessive atrophy, in particular, can increase the risk for bleeding.

POTENTIAL RISKS DURING DBS SURGERY

- Infection
- Bleeding
- Stroke
- Seizure
- Suboptimal placement of the DBS lead
- Coughing in the operating room (air embolism)

POTENTIAL SIDE EFFECTS THAT MAY EMERGE AFTER DBS SURGERY

- Infection
- Venous stroke
- Headache
- Confusion
- An electrically shorted or broken lead (fracture)
- Depression
- Anxiety
- Apathy
- Suicidality (suicidal thoughts, suicidal ideation)
- Hypomania or mania (increased moodiness, inability to sleep, racing thoughts)
- Impulse-control issues (gambling, shopping, hypersexuality)
- Dyskinesia (involuntary movements)
- Worsening walking and balance
- Trouble thinking
- Trouble speaking intended words (verbal fluency)

The past 10 to 20 years of DBS experience have provided a number of important lessons. The first is that aggressively reducing medication may result in apathy, depression, and other neuropsychological issues. Second, the original premise that DBS should replace medications has been revised. We now believe that the best outcomes following DBS surgery result from using an appropriate amount of medications in the short and long term. Commonly, medications are aggressively reduced following STN DBS in an effort to lessen stimulation-induced movements (such as dyskinesia). In many cases, this practice can result in apathy, depression, and worsening motor symptoms. In some cases, GPi DBS implants are used in patients who have "brittle dyskinesia." In brittle dyskinesia cases, patients experience the symptom of abnormal dance-like movements when taking low doses of Sinemet (one 25/100 tablet or less per dose). Using a GPi target for a brittle dyskinesia patient will facilitate more flexibility in medication adjustments, particularly later in the course of Parkinson's disease. The GPi target is rarely associated with stimulation-induced dyskinesias or dance-like movements.

Length of the Effects of DBS

One of the most commonly asked questions is whether the effects of DBS last forever. This is actually a complex question. The most important principle to remember in answering this question is that DBS has not been shown to stop disease progression (it is not neuroprotective). This means that the disease will continue to progress despite the DBS, and that walking, balance, talking, and thinking symptoms will be among the most prominent. The rigidity and bradykinesia (slowness of movement) will usually have longer-lasting improvements and, as long as the specific symptoms respond to the dopamine replacement therapy, these symptoms will continue to improve. We have been impressed by observing DBS patients who have had implants for 20 years, noting that tremor, motor fluctuations, and involuntary movements (dyskinesia) remain improved in the long term.

WHAT TYPE OF DEVICE SHOULD I CHOOSE?

Now that multiple devices are FDA-approved (Medtronic, Abbott, and Boston Scientific), we frequently see the same mistake continue to play out—choosing the device prior to the multidisciplinary screening. We suggest a sequence of steps that begins with a multidisciplinary screening, followed by a review of the FDA approval and specific target, then, finally, consideration of the features of each device. Patients and families should also be aware that a technology race is ongoing, and many features will be added to devices through both hardware and software improvements.

We recommend the following six tips for clinicians when they are choosing a specific device for individual patients:

Tip 1 — Make a determination of disease, the optimal brain target(s), and the approach (unilateral vs. bilateral), as this may narrow the choice of device.

Tip 2 — Assess access to programming and technical support for the device.

Tip 3 — Keep in mind that a rechargeable device is not always the best option.

Tip 4 — Decide on the likelihood that full-body MRI imaging will be needed in future.

Tip 5 — Decide on the need for current steering or current shaping.

Tip 6 — Choose a programming platform that you are experienced and comfortable with using in the office.

Focused Ultrasound Therapy

Conventional DBS therapy involves drilling a dime-sized hole in the skull and inserting a lead to record physiology (e.g., microelectrode) as well as permanent leads directly into the brain target or region. A similar procedure is used for mapping the brain before surgery that places a destructive lesion (thalamotomy, subthalamotomy, and pallidotomy). Recently, an alternative, ultrasound-based approach has been gaining popularity. High-intensity ultrasound was introduced in the 1940s and 1950s as a treatment for a variety of brain disorders. Its recent rebirth has generated much enthusiasm and excitement, and has included combining ultrasound with high-field MRI scanning.

Ultrasound therapy for essential tremor and Parkinson's disease has great appeal to patients and families. It does not require a scalp incision or drilling a hole in the skull. Additionally, the therapy has several advantages over gamma knife and other radiosurgical techniques. In radiosurgery, the surgeon aims X-ray beams at the brain and destroys tissue. In ultrasound, the tissue is still destroyed, but there is an option to apply a test-lesion prior to placing a permanent one. Another disadvantage of radiation therapy, when compared to ultrasound, is that the X-rays can lead to necrosis (dying) and uncontrolled growth of radiation-induced brain lesions. These lesions can, in some cases, expand uncontrollably in size, leading to delayed complications and, in one case, resulting in a death.

Considerations for Ultrasound Therapy

- Ultrasound is FDA-approved as a therapy for Parkinson's disease, but only in one target area of the brain (the VIM thalamic target), which will only treat the tremor, not the other symptoms of Parkinson's disease.
- The risks of ultrasound are similar to the risks of placing a conventional brain lesion (thalamotomy, subthalamotomy, and pallidotomy), with the exception of decreased infection rate because there is no permanent hardware placed.

- Since a destructive brain lesion can be created with both ultrasound and conventional thalamotomy (placing a heated probe into the brain), patients should be careful to not be misled by ultrasound marketing that sometimes uses the word "scalpel-less." While it is true that no scalpel is used and no incision is made, patients should not be deceived into thinking this procedure is without risk. Although the surgical risks (such as infection) are eliminated, the therapeutic effect of this intervention is achieved by destroying brain tissue. If the destructive lesion is not limited to the intended target, permanent neurological deficits may occur, as they can with conventional surgery (thalamotomy).
- A bilateral or two-sided ultrasound brain surgery (operating on both the right and left brain) is discouraged because of a high potential for side effects (such as cognition, swallowing, and speech). This limitation can be a serious issue and a risk for Parkinson's disease patients who may require two-sided surgery because of disabling symptoms on both sides of their body.
- Microelectrode recording and physiological mapping cannot be used to refine brain targets in ultrasound therapy.
- Precision of placement of the ultrasound lesion has been a big hurdle and will require refinement, especially as trials are conducted in Parkinson's disease patients. Patients should be educated that the ultrasound wave is generated outside of the skull, and, because it comes from outside the skull, this creates a formidable challenge for millimeter-sized targets deep within the brain. The technology and experience continue to improve.
- One benefit of ultrasound therapy (similar to pallidotomy, subthalamotomy, or thalamotomy) is that, after the procedure, there are no wires, pacemakers, or follow-up visits for programming or optimization.
- Ultrasound therapy is not a cure for Parkinson's disease.

A Concluding Note on Ultrasound Therapy

The bottom line for patients is that ultrasound therapy is scalpel-less, and it is not a cure. In the future, it may become more prominent as a treatment for Parkinson's disease, but in the meantime, patients should ensure they are aware of its potential benefits and risks. It may be ideal for those patients for whom tremor is the only bothersome symptom, and it could be useful in the elderly, who are at high risk for conventional DBS or lesion-based surgery (for example, for patients on blood thinners). Finally, ultrasound is approved only for the one target in the brain (thalamic), and this brain location is rarely utilized in modern Parkinson's disease surgery.

PEARLS FOR A BETTER LIFE

SURGICAL THERAPIES FOR PARKINSON'S DISEASE

*I have made many mistakes myself; I have spoiled
a hatful; the best surgeon, like the best general,
is he who makes the fewest mistakes.*
— SIR ASTLEY PASTON COOPER

➤ When selecting a surgical team, experience matters.

➤ Not everyone should receive deep brain stimulation (DBS) or other surgical therapies.

➤ The best scenario you can hope for is to be evaluated by a DBS multidisciplinary team who "talk behind your back" and plan every aspect of your surgery and aftercare.

➤ DBS surgery is not one-size-fits-all, and the brain target, approach (unilateral versus bilateral), and staging (one procedure or several) can make the difference between success and failure.

➤ The DBS lead location cannot be determined by imaging alone (CT or MRI) but is also determined by programming.

➤ The most critical element of DBS outcome after proper selection is location, location, location (of the DBS lead). No amount of expert programming can make up for a misplaced DBS lead.

➤ Once an adequate DBS setting is chosen, there are usually minimal if any programming changes over time. This is in contrast to medications and other therapies, which are in constant flux following DBS surgery.

- More important than DBS programming is monitoring and treating the neuropsychiatric and other aspects of the Parkinson's disease.

- DBS surgery is not a cure.

- The symptoms most likely to improve with DBS are tremor, rigidity, bradykinesia, off time, on-off fluctuations, and dyskinesia.

- Walking, talking, and thinking are usually not improved by DBS surgery.

- The choice of DBS device should occur as the last step in the multidisciplinary discussion. The device choice should be tailored as much as possible to your individual needs.

- All devices, regardless of manufacturer, will work well if optimally placed within the brain.

- Though radiosurgery and focused ultrasound are "incisionless," a permanent hole is still placed in the brain.

- Radiosurgery and focused ultrasound are therapies directed at the target from outside the brain. These therapies do not use physiological guidance or microelectrode recording.

- Radiosurgery, focused ultrasound, or conventional lesion surgery (pallidotomy, thalamotomy, subthalamotomy) should not be performed on both sides of the brain.

- Radiosurgery (gamma knife) has delayed benefits and delayed side effects, and the radiation damage can slowly spread into unintended brain areas.

- Ultrasound therapy has fewer infections and fewer bleeds.

- Brain lesion therapy should not be performed on both sides of the brain as it can lead to irreversible talking and thinking problems.

SELECTED REFERENCES

Bronstein JM, Tagliati M, Alterman RL, Lozano AM, Volkmann J, Stefani A, Horak FB, Okun MS, Foote KD, Krack P, Pahwa R, Henderson JM, Hariz MI, Bakay RA, Rezai A, Marks WJ Jr, Moro E, Vitek JL, Weaver FM, Gross RE, DeLong MR. Deep brain stimulation for Parkinson disease: an expert consensus and review of key issues. *Archives of Neurology*, 2011 Feb;68(2):165.

Mikos A, Zahodne L, Okun MS, Foote K, Bowers D. Cognitive declines after unilateral deep brain stimulation surgery in Parkinson's disease: a controlled study using Reliable Change, part II. *Clinical Neuropsychologist*, 2010 Feb;24(2):235–45.

Okun MS. Tips for choosing a deep brain stimulation device. *JAMA Neurology*, 2019 Jul 1;76(7):749–50.

Okun MS. Deep-brain stimulation—entering the era of human neural-network modulation. *New England Journal of Medicine*, 2014 Oct 9;371(15):1369–73.

Okun MS. Deep-brain stimulation for Parkinson's disease. *New England Journal of Medicine*, 2012 Oct 18;367(16):1529–38.

Okun MS, Fernandez HH, Wu SS, Kirsch-Darrow L, Bowers D, Bova F, Suelter M, Jacobson CE 4th, Wang X, Gordon CW Jr, Zeilman P, Romrell J, Martin P, Ward H, Rodriguez RL, Foote KD. Cognition and mood in Parkinson's disease in subthalamic nucleus versus globus pallidus interna deep brain stimulation: the COMPARE trial. *Annals of Neurology*, 2009 May;65(5):586–95.

Okun MS, Foote KD. Parkinson's disease DBS: what, when, who and why? The time has come to tailor DBS targets. *Expert Review of Neurotherapeutics*, 2010 Dec;10(12):1847–57.

Okun MS, Foote KD. Subthalamic nucleus vs globus pallidus interna deep brain stimulation, the rematch: will pallidal deep brain stimulation make a triumphant return? *Archives of Neurology*, 2005 Apr;62(4):533–36.

Schuepbach WM, Rau J, Knudsen K, Volkmann J, Krack P, Timmermann L, Hälbig TD, Hesekamp H, Navarro SM, Meier N, Falk D, Mehdorn M, Paschen S, Maarouf M, Barbe MT, Fink GR, Kupsch A, Gruber D, Schneider GH, Seigneuret E, Kistner A, Chaynes P, Ory-Magne F, Brefel Courbon C, Vesper J, Schnitzler A, Wojtecki L, Houeto JL, Bataille B, Maltête D, Damier P, Raoul S, Sixel-Doering F, Hellwig D, Gharabaghi A, Krüger R, Pinsker MO, Amtage F, Régis JM, Witjas T, Thobois S, Mertens P, Kloss M, Hartmann A, Oertel WH, Post B, Speelman H, Agid Y, Schade-Brittinger C, Deuschl G; EARLYSTIM Study Group. Neurostimulation for Parkinson's disease with early motor complications. *New England Journal of Medicine*, 2013 Feb 14;368(7):610–22.

Wagle Shukla A, Okun MS. Surgical treatment of Parkinson's disease: patients, targets, devices, and approaches. *Neurotherapeutics*, 2014 Jan;11(1):47–59.

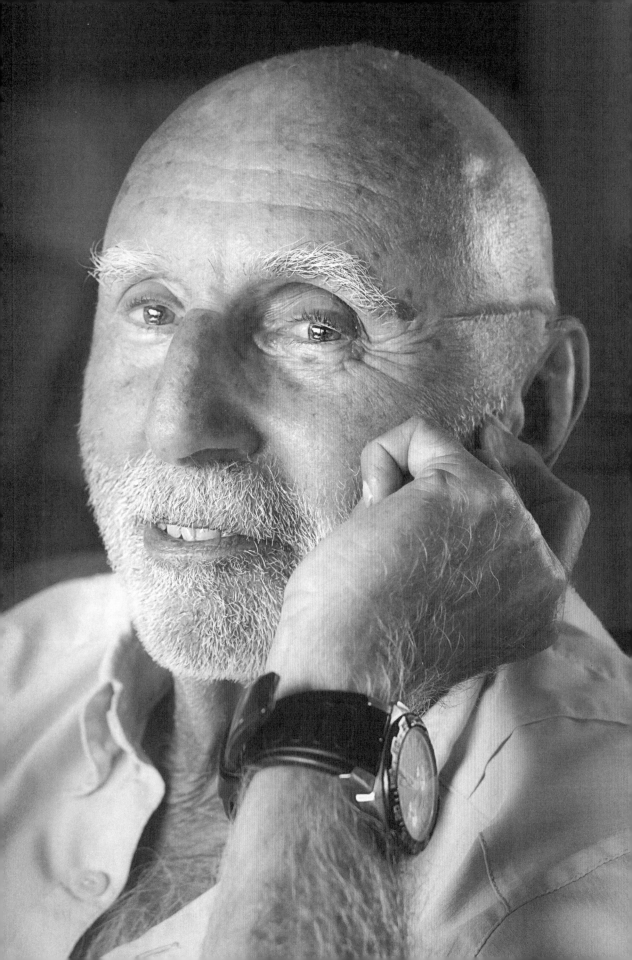

CHAPTER 7

NUTRITION AND THE MICROBIOME

**If you don't take care of your body,
where are you going to live?
– Unknown author**

FOOD PASSES THROUGH multiple body parts, which, together, form what is known as the gastrointestinal (GI) tract. The process starts as food passes from the mouth down to the stomach by way of the esophagus, then enters the small intestine. Once past multiple sections of the small intestine, food passes through the large intestine, then, finally, out the rectum and anus, where food waste (called stool) is released. The surface area of the GI tract is estimated to be half the size of a badminton court (440 square feet). This large surface area facilitates digestion of food and absorption of nutrients. Billions of bacteria and other beneficial microbes live in the GI tract and help digest and absorb food.

In Chapter 5, we discussed in detail the different parts of the GI tract that can be affected by Parkinson's disease, such as slowing of the stomach (gastroparesis), which can lead to indigestion and irregular medication absorption. There can also be slowness of the movement of the small intestines, resulting in indigestion and bloating. And, finally, there can be slowness of movements of the colon, resulting in constipation. In this chapter, we discuss a number of Parkinson's disease symptoms and how they relate to nutrition and the microbiome.

Dysphagia

Dysphagia (swallowing difficulty) is common in Parkinson's disease. More than 80 percent of individuals with Parkinson's disease will develop some element of dysphagia. It is usually found in the more advanced stages of Parkinson's disease, but it can occur early in the disease. Dysphagia can lead to multiple complications, such as aspiration pneumonia, malnutrition, and dehydration (due to reduced intake of foods and fluids). Parkinson's disease reduces saliva production, especially in the "OFF" medication state, which may worsen dysphagia. Salivary production improves in many patients when in the "ON" medication state. Parkinson's disease patients have a slower drinking rate and frequently drink a smaller volume at a time when compared to individuals without Parkinson's disease. An evaluation by a speech and swallowing therapist—using multiple X-rays to observe how different consistencies of solid or liquid foods are swallowed—can help identify a potential swallowing problem.

If swallowing problems are identified, modifications to food and/or liquid intake are recommended. For example, in a study involving 40 participants, 87 percent had an improvement of their swallowing function when they were administered carbonated liquids. More evaluations of alternative strategies to improve swallowing are critically needed. A swallowing test is recommended for individuals at a more advanced stage of the disease (three and above on the Hoehn & Yahr scale), for those with a history of coughing while eating or drinking, or for those with self-reported swallowing problems.

→ **CLINICAL PEARL**

Coughing while eating or experiencing food "sticking" in the throat are important signs for patients and caregivers to recognize. If these symptoms occur, an evaluation by a speech and swallowing therapist should be considered.

Constipation

Constipation is common in Parkinson's disease and it is one of the most common complaints we hear in our clinical practice. Many people tell us that they had problems with constipation years before being diagnosed with Parkinson's disease. Constipation is not only infrequent bowel movements (fewer than three per week), but also bowel movements that require straining or that feel incomplete. The normal pattern of bowel movements can and will vary by one to three days. A stool-voiding pattern of every day or every other day is encouraged. Constipation can result in poor appetite, indigestion, bloating, and worsening motor function. Higher levodopa dosages are required for individuals with constipation, independent of disease duration. Having a fiber-rich diet and ensuring adequate hydration are important strategies to improve this symptom. The vast majority of adults do not meet fiber recommendations. Our patients are encouraged to eat two to three cups of fruit, two to three cups of vegetables, and three to six ounces of whole grains each day. Legumes (beans, peas, and lentils) should also be consumed at least three times per week.

Using over-the-counter stool softeners and laxatives can be helpful in management of constipation. These products should be used infrequently, as they can have side effects, including dependency. Diet modification, adequate hydration, and increasing your level of physical activity should be tried before regularly including laxatives or stool softeners.

→ CLINICAL PEARL

Increasing intake of fiber from fruits, vegetables, whole grains, and legumes with adequate hydration may aid in management of constipation. Smoothies are a great way to incorporate more fiber into your diet. Adding a couple of handfuls of baby spinach to your favorite smoothie significantly increases your fiber intake.

Causes of Constipation

There are many possible causes of constipation in Parkinson's disease. These include the following.

Change in Activity/Lowered Activity

Exercise and increased activity will assist in establishing regular bowel patterns.

Change in Diet/Low-Fiber Diet

An ideal diet will include fiber-rich foods such as bran, whole-grain breads and cereals, oatmeal, pasta, nuts, popcorn, brown rice, fruits, vegetables, beans, peas, and lentils.

Medical Reasons

Cancer, pregnancy, hemorrhoids, neurological disorder, muscular disorder, and intestinal inflammation can cause constipation.

Medications

NSAIDs, narcotics, sedatives, antacids, antispasmodics, and iron supplements can cause constipation.

BOWEL CLEAN OUT

The bowel clean out should be done before starting on the bowel program that is outlined for you by your physician. This should be done on a day when you will be at home all day, to minimize the risk of accidentally soiling your clothes. The bowel clean out is a two-part procedure:

1. In the morning take two ounces of magnesium hydroxide (e.g., Milk of Magnesia) and follow that with a hot drink, such as hot coffee, hot tea, or even hot broth. This helps stimulate the bowel.

2. The same evening, after dinner, give yourself a saline enema (e.g., Fleet). This helps make sure the rectum is empty. You should be able to rest the night without worry or discomfort.

This procedure may be repeated the next day if needed.

A NATURAL CONSTIPATION STRATEGY

When daily vigorous exercise and drinking six to eight glasses of water per day has not worked, we often share the following recipe (refined by Janet Romrell, a physician assistant in our practice):

- 1 cup unprocessed wheat bran
- ½ cup apple sauce
- ½ cup prune juice

Mix the ingredients together and refrigerate. Replace the mixture each week. Take one to two tablespoons daily for one week for desired results. If needed, increase dose by one tablespoon each week. Stool frequency and gas may increase the first few weeks but will usually adjust after one month.

You can also sprinkle bran on food to supplement your fiber intake. The minimum amount of fiber that is recommended each day is approximately 25 grams, but you may require more, depending on your age and stage of Parkinson's disease.

Note: Unprocessed wheat bran can be purchased at most large grocery stores and is found with either the hot cereals or flours and baking goods. It can also be purchased in bulk at health food stores.

Not Drinking Enough Fluids

At least six to eight 8oz glasses of fluids per day is recommended. This includes everything a patient drinks (water, tea, coffee, juice, colas, etc.), but water is best and should be primary. Bladder patients should reduce fluid intake after the evening meal.

Medications to Manage Constipation

Here are some of the medication treatment options for constipation in Parkinson's disease.

Bulk Producing (Metamucil, FiberCon, or Citrucel)

Mix one to two tablespoons in juice or water and take by mouth, one to two times daily. This adds consistency or bulk to the stool and facilitates water retention in stool. (Patients must take adequate fluids by mouth to avoid causing constipation.)

Stool Softeners (Colace)

This softens stool by facilitating the mixture of fat and water. Stool softeners should not be used with mineral oil. Take one tablet by mouth, one to two times daily.

Combinations (Pericolace)

This is a mild stool softener and laxative combined. Take by mouth, one to two times daily.

Irritant/Stimulant (Products Containing Senna)

These are laxatives with direct action on the intestine and the bowel.

Suppositories (Glycerin, Dulcolax)

These are inserted rectally every other day or when needed. Suppositories stimulate the rectum and assist with evacuation.

Osmotic Laxative (Miralax)

This is a laxative used to treat constipation by increasing the amount of water in the stool. Bowel movements become easier and more frequent. Take as directed on the bottle (one dose is about one heaping tablespoon, added to 4 to 8oz of water, juice, soda, coffee, or tea, mixed well. Do not take more often than directed.

Probiotics (Phillips' Colon Health, Activia Yogurt)

Although these may be used for managing constipation, few probiotic supplements have been scientifically shown to help with constipation.

Weight Gain and Loss

Problems with the GI tract can lead to nutritional problems and can result in weight changes. Those with Parkinson's disease tend to experience weight fluctuations throughout the course of the disease. For most people, there is an initial loss of weight prior to diagnosis or even with the onset of the motor symptoms. Then, there is usually weight gain in the first few years after the diagnosis, followed by a steady and significant slow weight loss during subsequent years. The reason for the fluctuations in body weight are not clear and can be related to changes in the level of physical activity and to the development of motor fluctuations (such as dyskinesia).

A COMMON PATTERN OF WEIGHT CHANGES IN PARKINSON'S DISEASE

Before motor symptoms or diagnosis, weight loss is observed. Then, early in the disease, weight gain occurs, followed in the more advanced stages by steady and progressive weight loss. In these stages, sometimes increasing calorie intake does not stop the weight loss.

Malnutrition

Malnutrition in Parkinson's disease is a concern that has been underrecognized and underappreciated. It has been documented that malnutrition may be present in up to 24 percent of patients with Parkinson's disease, while 60 percent remain at risk. There is a correlation between malnutrition and markers of disease severity, and improvements in nutritional status may increase quality of life. There are several factors that increase the risk of malnutrition, including symptoms associated with decreased food intake and increased metabolism, living alone, mood problems, and older age at the time of diagnosis. Malnutrition can also occur with a higher amount of levodopa, although it is not clear if the higher levodopa dose is causing weight loss or is a sign of a more advanced disease that is associated with weight loss. Most experts believe the latter is true.

Often, patients with the highest risk for malnutrition tell us they do not feel hungry anymore, or they feel full quickly during meals. In both cases, eating six to eight small meals throughout the day may allow for greater overall nutritional intake. It can be helpful to focus on consuming calorie- and protein-dense foods to ensure adequate nutrition for each bite of food. For this reason, we encourage increasing foods from sources of healthy fats (e.g., extra-virgin olive oil, avocado) and proteins (e.g., yogurt, legumes, eggs, fatty fish, lean poultry, and meat). In some cases, patients may benefit from high-calorie, high-protein oral nutrition supplements (Ensure and Boost are examples) to help meet their nutritional needs. Many patients seem to get "out of the practice" of eating and thus their body comes to expect less food. With a little effort and a well-planned routine, a patient can learn to feel hungry again.

Weight loss and malnutrition are associated with worsening of motor control and motor fluctuations (and an increased risk of falling), as well as decline in the quality of life. To decrease the risk of weight changes, an individual with Parkinson's disease and their caregiver should be proactive. This strategy should include tracking weight and nutrition regularly and identifying factors that can worsen nutrition and weight control. A consultation with a dietitian is helpful in monitoring and planning.

Beneficial Diets for Parkinson's Disease

One very common question is: "What is the best Parkinson's disease diet?" But there is no single correct answer. People with Parkinson's disease and their caregivers have different opinions about the diet that has worked best. Some insist on the benefits of a plant-based diet, some on the benefits of the Mediterranean diet, and others advocate for a ketogenic (low carbohydrate) diet. A recent study has correlated dietary patterns with Parkinson's disease progression. Food choices shown with potential benefits (for slower disease progression) were in keeping with the Mediterranean diet, which is high in fruits (in particular, blueberries, blackberries, strawberries, and raspberries), vegetables, whole grains, pulses, nuts, fatty fish (salmon, tuna, sardines, mackerel, and herring), and extra-virgin olive oil. The Mediterranean diet is also low in red meat (beef and pork) and low in refined sugar.

There is limited evidence that caffeinated coffee consumption is associated with a decreased risk of developing Parkinson's disease (although how and why is not clear). It has been suggested that specific mutations in a gene coding for a brain receptor may offer clues as to why some diets and products may possibly decrease the risk of developing Parkinson's disease and, in some cases, improve symptoms for existing sufferers. Certain types of milk have also been suggested as risk factors for the later development of Parkinson's disease.

It is important to remember that there are ongoing studies that are trying to determine if specific diets may offer advantages. There is no scientific consensus on the "ideal" diet for a patient with Parkinson's disease. It is not clear if there are dietary patterns associated with a higher risk of developing or worsening Parkinson's symptoms and there is no evidence suggesting that diet changes disease outcome. Hence, current diet recommendations rely on general health recommendations and there may be specific modifications related to accompanying symptoms (e.g., increasing fiber to help in the management of constipation).

THE CASE FOR A PLANT-BASED DIET

One hypothesis advocates for the use of a plant-based (vegetarian) diet. The rationale for this hypothesis is based on the idea that plants offer a large number of chemicals (called "phytochemicals") that have antioxidant properties, and that these may decrease inflammation, which is often associated with the changes in the brain observed in patients with Parkinson's disease. This remains unproven and studies are needed.

To Eat Protein or Not to Eat Protein

When a person with Parkinson's disease uses levodopa, pharmacists, doctors, and even friends frequently warn that consuming protein foods will make levodopa less effective, and that levodopa should not be combined with meals. The standard recommendation is to take levodopa 30 to 60 minutes before a meal or to wait one to two hours after meals.

The timing of medications relative to food intake, however, poses no concerns early in the disease course. At this stage, if a patient takes levodopa medication only three times per day, timing of meals may not affect absorption of the medications. As the disease progresses, a levodopa dose may be required more frequently (e.g., every two hours), and this may increase interaction around meal times.

If levodopa is being taken every two hours, timing the medication 30 to 45 minutes before a meal may be an optimal strategy. The recommendation for timing of this medication before meals is based on a previous study published in 2010 in the *Journal of Neurology*. Specifically, meals that contain protein may have an impact on the stomach emptying, and therefore may compete with absorption in the small intestine.

Levodopa is absorbed rapidly when consumed on an empty stomach and delay in the stomach emptying (due to the presence of protein foods) can interfere with the rate at which levodopa is absorbed. In addition, proteins are broken down into amino acids, which can compete with levodopa for absorption because of their similar chemical structures. Combining levodopa with a meal, particularly a protein-rich meal, may lead to a worsening of symptom control and the emergence of motor fluctuations. For those unable to tolerate taking levodopa on an empty stomach (due to nausea, for example), we usually recommend taking the medication with a simple carbohydrate (such as half a cup of 100-percent fruit juice), as this likely will not delay the stomach emptying or interfere with medication absorption.

Despite the potential concern of worsening Parkinson's symptoms if levodopa is taken with meals, for most people, this is not a major issue and they do not notice any significant motor fluctuations related to meal or medication timing. The small number of Parkinson's disease patients who may notice medication fluctuations seem to be at a high risk for protein-calorie malnutrition. Malnutrition may result from a drastic decrease in the amount of protein in the diet.

To avoid protein-calorie malnutrition, a protein redistribution diet can be trialed: The patient can restrict protein consumption during breakfast and lunch, but unrestrict protein consumption at dinner. This strategy, if not executed properly, can lead to protein-calorie malnutrition and has not been studied long-term or extensively in older individuals. Any protein restriction

The recommended daily protein intake is 0.8–1g for every kilogram of body weight. For example, a 70-year-old man weighing 80kg (176 lbs) and exercising moderately (four to five times per week) should consume between 64g and 80g of protein per day (equivalent to three servings of chicken breast).

recommendation should be reviewed with a doctor and dietitian. We usually recommend a consultation with a dietitian to ensure appropriate protein intake, as the amount needed may be affected by multiple factors, such as age, kidney disease, and level of exercise.

Supplements for a Parkinson's Disease Diet

There is significant evidence that Parkinson's disease is associated with increased inflammation and an imbalance of antioxidants (oxidative stress). Studies that have explored the use of antioxidants have not revealed positive benefits for Parkinson's disease. One critique of these studies was that, by the time Parkinson's disease symptoms are apparent, there is already too much accumulated damage.

The use of antioxidants prior to the onset of Parkinson's disease has been proposed as possibly offering more benefits, but few studies have evaluated the use of antioxidants prior to motor symptom onset and, further, there is a need for long-term follow-up for these studies to provide adequate evidence. Studies that have followed individuals with Parkinson's disease have provided conflicting results, with some study participants showing a possible decrease in the risk of developing Parkinson's disease when taking more antioxidants (such as vitamins C, E, and beta carotene), while other studies contradict these findings.

→ CLINICAL PEARL

There is no evidence that taking antioxidant supplements improves the symptoms of Parkinson's disease. We need more studies to help us know if there is any effect of supplements containing antioxidants.

Some of the nutritional problems in Parkinson's disease seem to be related to medication side effects. Many of the medications utilized (e.g., levodopa) can be associated with gastrointestinal side effects, such as nausea, stomach upset, and change in the taste of food. Additionally, levodopa can be associated with lower levels of certain vitamins, such as folic acid, vitamin B_6, and vitamin B_{12}. Low levels of these vitamins can, in select cases, result in neuropathy (nerve injury causing tingling and numbness) and the elevation of another compound (homocysteine), which at high levels increases the risk for heart disease. Vitamin supplements are usually recommended, although it is not clear if this will help decrease the risk of complications. Also, taking too much of some of the vitamin supplements (e.g., B_6) may result in neurological side effects such as neuropathy. One study suggests that vitamin D may slow Parkinson's disease progression in a small and specific group of individuals. Monitoring vitamin D levels and adding a supplement may be beneficial.

→ **CLINICAL PEARL**

Microbes in the intestines play an important role in regulating inflammation in the body.

Microbes in the intestines interact with the brain. Evidence strongly suggests that people with Parkinson's disease have an alteration in their intestinal microbes. It is not yet clear how to intervene or how to modify these microbes, or if modification will have any effect on the development or the improvement of Parkinson's disease symptoms. Ongoing research in this area may provide insight into how to manage symptoms through changing the gut microbiome.

A Concluding Note on the Microbiome In Parkinson's Disease

The gut microbiome consists of a diverse community of bacteria, fungi, and viruses (known as "microbes") that reside in the GI tract. There is increased interest in the role of these microbes, as they can have beneficial (or pathogenic) roles for human health. The presence and function of microbes can be influenced by a number of factors, including age, sex, environment, diet, and the use of medications and supplements. More recently, research published in 2015 in the *World Journal of Gastroenterology* and in 2017 in the *Journal of Cellular Physiology* showed there is bidirectional communication between the central nervous system and the GI system, which is referred to as the "gut-brain axis." Microbes interact with the nervous system in a variety of ways, such as (1) regulating inflammation; (2) producing neurotransmitters (chemical signals) such as dopamine and serotonin; and (3) influencing communication with the brain, which can affect the function of the GI tract and may influence behavior, mood, and memory function. The composition of the gut microbes may be different in patients with Parkinson's disease as compared to healthy individuals. Knowledge of how specific gut microbes influence the nervous system is ongoing and more research is needed to better understand them.

Diet is known to influence the gut microbiome by altering the composition of microbes along the GI tract. Beneficial microbes can play an important role in maintaining immune and GI function, maintaining integrity of the intestinal barrier, and maintaining healthy levels of prebiotic fibers. Prebiotic fibers can be naturally found in foods such as bananas, oats, onions, leeks, garlic, and asparagus. In addition, they are added to food products like yogurts and cereal bars. Recent research has found that a Mediterranean diet is associated with increased levels of beneficial bacteria, possibly due to increased fermentation of fibers from plant foods.

Prebiotic fibers can stimulate growth of probiotics, a live microorganism that can provide health benefits. Probiotics are commonly found in supplements, as additives and preservatives, and are used to create food products such as yogurt and cheese. Probiotics may have varied effects on health, including gastrointestinal health (constipation, diarrhea, irritable bowel diseases) and immunity. A 2017 study published in the journal *Gut*, for example, investigated the effect of probiotics and prebiotics in patients with Parkinson's disease who experience constipation. Researchers found that drinking a fermented milk containing a prebiotic and multiple strains of probiotic bacteria was associated with improving symptoms of constipation in this population.

The possible effects of lifestyle on the microbiome has received considerable interest, especially in regard to smoking and caffeine consumption. One hypothesis to explain the observed reduction in Parkinson's disease with caffeine consumption and cigarette smoking has been that they have been associated with changes in the gut microbes. Further work is required to evaluate the role of the gut microbes in the development and symptoms of Parkinson's disease, and further research is needed into strategies to manipulate these microbes.

NUTRITION AND THE MICROBIOME

*Our bodies are our gardens and
our wills are our gardeners.*
— WILLIAM SHAKESPEARE

➻ There is increasing evidence that there is a gut-brain connection in Parkinson's disease.

➻ The common gastrointestinal bug *H. pylori* affects approximately half of the world's population, and it can affect absorption of Parkinson's disease medications.

➻ Early research has revealed the possibility that certain diets (e.g., the Mediterranean diet) may be helpful in prevention and treatment of degenerative diseases.

➻ Probiotics and other nutritional approaches are promising; however, their effects across the Parkinson's disease population remain unknown.

➻ Foods, especially those containing protein, can influence absorption of Parkinson's disease medications.

➻ The majority of people with Parkinson's disease do not need to change their diet to improve medication absorption.

➻ The most common strategy to improve medication absorption is to give your medications a half hour head start before you eat.

➻ If you love wine or alcohol, the safest way to consume it is in small quantities—pouring just enough in the bottom of the glass to allow taste without impairment.

SELECTED REFERENCES

Contin M, Martinelli P. Pharmacokinetics of levodopa. *Journal of Neurology*, 2010 Nov;257:S253–61.

De Filippis F, Pellegrini N, Vannini L, Jeffery IB, La Storia A, Laghi L, Serrazanetti DI, Di Cagno R, Ferrocino I, et al. High-level adherence to a Mediterranean diet beneficially impacts the gut microbiota and associated metabolome. *Gut*, 2016;65:1812–21.

Food and Agriculture Organization of the United Nations, World Health Organization. *Guidelines for the Evaluation of Probiotics*, 2002.

Mulak A, Bonaz B. Brain-gut-microbiota axis in Parkinson's disease. *World Journal of Gastroenterology*, 2015 Oct 7;21:10609–20.

Mittal R, Debs LH, Patel AP, Nguyen D, Patel K, O'Connor G, Grati M, Mittal J, Yan D, et al. Neurotransmitters: the critical modulators regulating gut-brain axis. *Journal of Cellular Physiology*, 2017 Sep;232:2359–72.

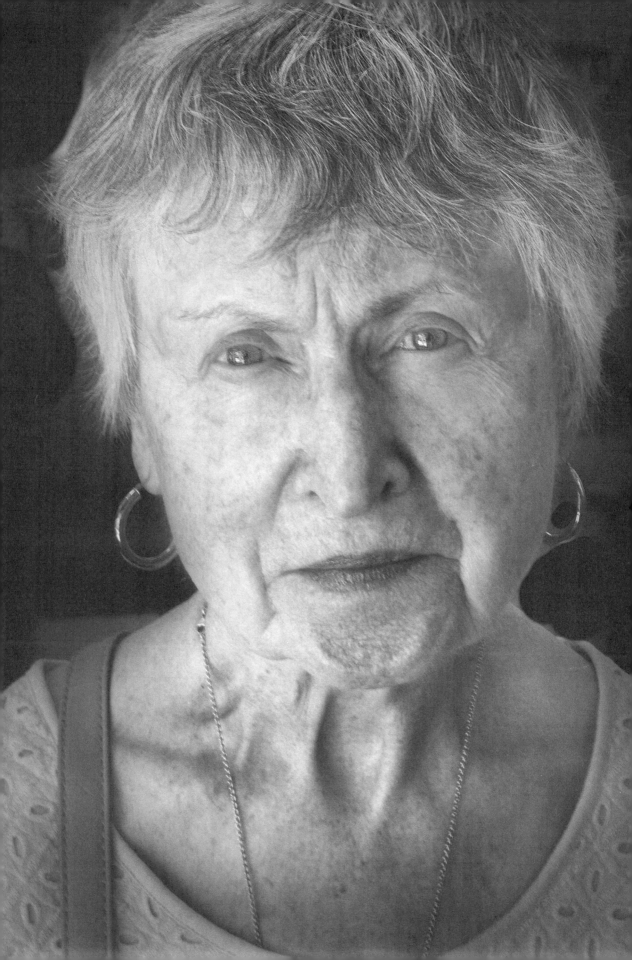

CHAPTER 8

TREATMENT OF NEUROPSYCHIATRIC PARKINSON'S DISEASE SYMPTOMS

*At times, I feel overwhelmed and
my depression leads me into darkness.*
– Dorothy Hamill

ALTHOUGH THE PARKINSON'S DISEASE motor symptoms are the most recognizable, they are not always the greatest source of distress. In fact, 2018 research published in the *Journal of Korean Medical Science* showed that depression and anxiety can have the strongest influence on quality of life for someone with Parkinson's disease. Although tremor and falling can be disruptive, mood and psychological factors can result in an equally significant (or even more significant) impairment. Recognizing and treating depression and other disorders of mood, motivation, and thinking is a critical part of wellness in Parkinson's disease. In this chapter, we will discuss treatment of depression, anxiety, cognitive changes, apathy, and psychosis.

Depression

Experiencing depression is common in Parkinson's disease. Although major depressive disorder affects about one in five people with Parkinson's disease, if we expand this to include minor depression and depressive symptoms, about 35 percent of people with Parkinson's disease will have clinically significant depression at some point in their illness. This can occur very early and even before outward signs of Parkinson's disease. It can also occur later in the disease course.

Symptoms of Depression

→ **CLINICAL PEARL**

Minor depression occurs when you have a few symptoms of depression but are still able to function. Major depression has been described as a low or depressed mood and/or loss of interest and pleasure in usual activities. There may also be other symptoms.

According to the *Diagnostic and Statistical Manual of Mental Disorders* (DSM-5) and clinical experience, the following are the symptoms of depression:

- Sad or depressed mood that persists on most days
- Easy tearfulness
- Feeling hopeless or defeated
- Changes in sleep patterns (too little or too much)
- Loss of interest in or ability to experience pleasure from things usually enjoyed
- Feelings of worthlessness or guilt that are excessive and frequent
- Reduced energy
- Persistent change in appetite (decrease or increase in appetite and weight loss or gain)
- Irritability and easy aggravation
- Problems with concentration and decisiveness
- Difficulty with memory

- Physical problems that cannot be explained by the patient's doctors
- Slowing down of thoughts or movements
- Recurrent thoughts of death or suicidal thoughts

DID YOU KNOW?

Some of these symptoms can be seen in Parkinson's disease even when a person is not depressed. Slowness, trouble thinking, and changes in appetite and sleep are examples. This can make it tricky to disentangle symptoms of Parkinson's disease in general from symptoms of untreated Parkinson's-related depression.

CASE EXAMPLE — GEORGE

George is a 61-year-old man who was diagnosed with Parkinson's disease at age 54. He takes carbidopa/levodopa (25/100, two pills, four times daily), but has been experiencing the wearing off between dosages and dyskinesia (uncontrolled, involuntary movement) 20 minutes after a dose "kicks in." He is reporting difficulty in working at his family-owned restaurant. He has experienced some "near misses," almost dropping trays he was carrying back and forth to the kitchen. He is up at night worrying about whether or not he will be able to continue working as long as he had previously planned. At home, he has feelings of guilt about how his wife has been performing more of the tasks he traditionally performed. He describes himself as feeling less joyful, even with activities that typically would give him a lot of pleasure. He has no interest in sexual activity. His wife notices he has less appetite and energy and is becoming progressively more isolated.

George sees his movement disorder specialist, who suspects depression and initiates a serotonin reuptake inhibitor (SSRI). At a six-week follow-up, George and his wife recognize that he has been feeling and acting more like "himself." He is dealing more effectively with stressors. He has resumed golfing on the weekends. He continues to feel sad in appropriate situations and he describes himself as happy during his daily life.

Treatment of Depression

Though treatable, depression in Parkinson's disease may be more difficult to treat than depression in the general population. This is because multiple chemicals in the brain, referred to as neurotransmitter systems, are involved. When depression is present, there are ongoing changes in the brain circuits that depend on two other brain chemicals, serotonin and norepinephrine. Many people forget that Parkinson's disease is much more than a dysfunction involving dopamine. In other words, depression in Parkinson's disease is not "just a dopamine problem" or "just a serotonin problem." Depression results from complex changes in the brain circuitry. The good news is that there are many treatments available and correcting the chemical imbalances can help improve symptoms. Here are a few of the most important treatment tips.

The Benefit Is Not Instant

It can take four to six weeks for antidepressants to take effect. After this time period has lapsed, if a benefit has not occurred or is incomplete, increasing the dose may be necessary. It is important to allow adequate time to experience the full benefit.

There Are Many Options

Too often, especially if there is a history of depression or anxiety that predates a Parkinson's disease diagnosis, medication trials for depression are too short or the dose is not high enough to have an impact on the symptoms. A side effect of one drug may result in fear of trying a different drug. It is important to know that there are many options, and not to give up after the first drug.

Each Patient Is Unique

Patients must avoid the temptation to draw conclusions from another person's experience with depression, which may involve factors that are specific to their case, including other health conditions, unique body chemistry, liver enzymes that metabolize the drugs, medication interactions, and individual disabling symptoms.

Consider a Blood Test

If multiple drugs and dosages fail to improve depression, a blood test may be useful. There is a condition in which depression medications are not being metabolized, but a simple blood test can reveal this problem and help lead to adequate treatment. In the near future, we may be more routinely using genetic testing to select the most effective medication for an individual (this field of research is called "pharmacogenomics").

Keep Trying

Expect trial and error in order to discover the best approach.

→ CLINICAL PEARL

Before treating depression, it is important to rule out any other explanation for changes in mood or behavior. Examples include underactive thyroid (which can result in low energy) and some medications, such as beta blockers (used for hypertension or heart conditions), which can mimic depression symptoms. Furthermore, it is a good idea to consult with your neurologist to be sure that Parkinson's disease medications are optimized, so that Parkinson's wellness is optimized and depression can be treated appropriately.

Sleep, Exercise, and Depression

Adequate sleep and physical exercise are important tools for managing depression. Exercise releases endorphins (natural brain opioids) that can boost mood and energy. Participating in a support group or community-based program (like boxing or cycling for Parkinson's disease) can in some cases improve Parkinson's disease. If opting for a support group, it is important to search for a group that is "compatible" with the desired level of activity and the stage of life. For example, individuals with young-onset Parkinson's disease can benefit from virtual or in-person groups tailored to their needs. We have been impressed in our practices to see that depression can in many cases lift when a patient discovers the right support network.

When depression requires treatment, in some cases, cognitive behavioral therapy (CBT) is useful. CBT requires meetings with a trained psychologist, to identify and analyze the contributors to depression, then uses techniques and develops strategies to change and overcome thought patterns or behaviors. It can be especially helpful when there are circumstances beyond the biological changes in brain chemicals that are having an impact on depression. For example, marital stressors, illness in friends or family, and difficulty in adjusting lifestyle may all be eased with CBT. Consulting a psychologist to process the challenges of a diagnosis and discuss treatment options can provide health benefits. Recent reviews of current treatment options for Parkinson's disease depression—published in *CNS Drugs* in 2018 and in *Movement Disorders* in 2019—revealed that CBT was likely effective, although this did not involve a large formal study in Parkinson's disease.

WHAT'S TRICKY ABOUT DIAGNOSING DEPRESSION IN PARKINSON'S DISEASE?

Some symptoms of depression, such as low energy and slowed movements, can be attributed to Parkinson's disease. The presence of these symptoms in patients with Parkinson's disease could result in missing a diagnosis of depression. At the same time, a person with Parkinson's disease may look "sad" or less expressive (poker-face), have a forward-flexed head (due to dystonia), and a flexed-forward change in posture. A person with Parkinson's disease may have less energy but may not always be depressed. These Parkinson's disease features may overlap with symptoms of depression. Expert assessment can help sort out the precise cause(s) of the symptoms.

→ CLINICAL PEARL

Because depression in Parkinson's disease is in large part biological and due to chemical changes in the brain, it is important to understand that depression is not just a reaction to circumstances. Medication or other therapies may be required to adequately treat the condition.

Depression Medications Used in Parkinson's Disease

There are several classes of medication that can be utilized in Parkinson's disease. The common thread between all of the medications is that they work to enhance the brain chemical serotonin and, in some cases, the brain chemical epinephrine.

Selective Serotonin Reuptake Inhibitors (SSRIs)

These work by slowing down the reabsorption of the brain chemical serotonin, thus making it more available in the brain. Common examples of SSRIs include fluoxetine, paroxetine, escitalopram, citalopram, and sertraline.

Selective Serotonin-Norepinephrine Reuptake Inhibitors (SNRIs)

These work in a manner similar to SSRIs, but also increase the brain chemical norepinephrine (thus the addition of the "N" to the name). Common examples include medications such as venlafaxine and duloxetine. SNRIs are also prescribed for pain relief in other conditions, such as back pain or neuropathy.

Tricyclic Antidepressants (TCAs)

This class of medications has a long history of use for depression and has been shown to be just as effective as SSRIs. Using a TCA, however, has many possible side effects that must be monitored, including dizziness, tiredness, confusion, hallucinations, urinary retention, constipation, and heart rhythm changes. Common examples of TCAs include nortriptyline and amitriptyline. At least one randomized study shows TCA versus SSRI producing similar results for Parkinson's disease depression. TCAs (like SSRIs) are sometimes used to manage pain, including headaches, back pain, and neuropathy.

Monoamine Oxidase Type B Inhibitors (MAO-B-Is)

This is an enzyme that breaks down serotonin and dopamine (both are "monoamine" neurotransmitters), which results in making serotonin and dopamine more available in the brain. Increasing serotonin is thought to have an antidepressant effect. The additional action of increasing dopamine facilitates mild improvement of the motor symptoms of Parkinson's disease. Some MAO-B inhibitors have important interactions with other medications (anaesthetics, pain medications, dextromethorphan), so it is important, when visiting the clinic, emergency room, or hospital, to ensure that doctors (particularly anesthesiologists) are aware that this is being taken. Low-dose MAO-B inhibitors are generally safe to take with antidepressants but should be monitored by a doctor.

Dopamine Agonists

Dopamine agonists are commonly prescribed for Parkinson's disease and have been reported to improve depression in some patients in addition to helping improve the motor symptoms. More information about dopamine agonists is available in Chapter 4.

Additional Treatment Considerations

Beyond oral medications (pills), a number of additional therapies have been administered to alleviate depression, including the following.

Repetitive Transcranial Magnetic Stimulation (rTMS)

Approved as a treatment for major depressive disorder, rTMS may be helpful for Parkinson's disease depression. It involves using a strong magnet to stimulate parts of the brain (dorsolateral prefrontal cortex) related to the depression circuits, which may influence communication with the deeper brain regions. Studies of this treatment in Parkinson's disease have had conflicting outcomes, so the full long-term impact is not yet known.

Electroconvulsive Therapy (ECT)

This method is utilized to treat severe medication refractory depression. It is a powerful therapy and, while patients and families may be reluctant to embrace it, it has a long-term safety record. Many experts describe the therapy as "resetting the software" of the brain. It may have side effects on memory and is considered only when psychiatrists have been involved and multiple other medical and behavioral therapies have been tried.

DID YOU KNOW?

Physical exercise has been shown to:

- Help motor symptoms of Parkinson's disease
- Improve balance and reduce falls
- Reduce depressive symptoms
- Improve sleep
- Help reduce progression of mild cognitive impairment toward more severe memory problems
- Support general health and "successful" aging

NOTE: Do not miss out on the benefits of physical exercise! Longer and more intense exercise seems to have the most benefit, but any level of physical activity is better than inactivity. Working with a physical therapist can help you find the best way to start.

COMMON DEPRESSION TREATMENTS

The following summary is provided courtesy of and with permission of the Parkinson's Foundation Mind, Mood, and Memory educational series.

MEDICATION (PRODUCT NAME IN PARENTHESES)	DOSAGES IN MILLIGRAMS (TABLETS UNLESS OTHERWISE NOTED)	TYPICAL TREATMENT REGIMENS	POTENTIAL SIDE EFFECTS	INDICATIONS FOR USAGE (ITALICS = APPROVED BY U.S. FDA)
Remember to discuss the risks of combined usage of antidepressants and the MAO-B inhibitors (selegiline or rasagiline) with your doctor				
SELECTIVE SEROTONIN REUPTAKE INHIBITORS (SSRIS)				
Citalopram (Celexa)	10, 20, 40mg tablets; 10mg/2ml solution	10–40mg daily	Headache, nausea, insomnia, vivid dreams, sedation, jitteriness, diminished sexual libido, weight gain	*Depression, anxiety/panic, obsessive-compulsive disorder (OCD)*
Escitalopram (Lexapro)	5, 10, 20mg tablets; 5mg/5ml solution	5–20mg daily	Same as above but weight neutral	*Depression, anxiety/panic, OCD*

MEDICATION (PRODUCT NAME IN PARENTHESES)	DOSAGES IN MILLIGRAMS (TABLETS UNLESS OTHERWISE NOTED)	TYPICAL TREATMENT REGIMENS	POTENTIAL SIDE EFFECTS	INDICATIONS FOR USAGE (ITALICS = APPROVED BY U.S. FDA)
Fluoxetine (Prozac)	10, 20, 40, 90	10–40 mg daily	Same as previous	*Depression, anxiety/panic, OCD*
Fluvoxamine (generic, Luvox CR)	25, 50, 100; CR 100, 150	25–100mg daily/nightly (may be different for extended release)	Headache, nausea, insomnia, vivid dreams, sedation, jitteriness, diminished sexual libido, weight gain	Depression, anxiety/panic, *OCD*
Paroxetine (Paxil, Paxil CR, Pexeva)	10, 12.5, 20, 25, 30, 37.5, 40mg tablets; 10mg/5ml suspension; CR 12.5 25, 37.5	10–40mg daily (may be different for extended release)	Same as above	*Depression, anxiety/panic, OCD*
Sertraline (Zoloft)	25, 50, 100mg tablets; 20mg/ml concentrate	25–100mg daily	Headache, nausea, insomnia, vivid dreams, sedation, jitteriness, diminished sexual libido, weight gain	*Depression, anxiety/panic, OCD*
Vilazodone	10, 20, 40	10–40 daily	Diarrhea, nausea, dizziness, dry mouth, insomnia, vomiting, vivid dreams	*Depression,* anxiety/panic, OCD

SEROTONIN-NOREPINEPHRINE REUPTAKE INHIBITORS (SNRIS)

Desvenlafaxine (Pristiq)	50, 100	50mg daily	Nausea, headache, insomnia, vivid dreams, sedation, jitteriness, dry mouth, constipation, diminished libido	*Depression,* anxiety
Duloxetine (Cymbalta)	20, 30, 60	10–30mg twice a day	Same as above	*Depression, anxiety*
Milnacipran (Savella)	12.5, 25, 50, 100	50mg twice per day	Same as above	Depression, anxiety
Nefazodone (Serzone)	50, 100, 150, 200, 250	25–100mg twice per day	Same as above, plus requires monitoring for liver function	*Depression,* anxiety

MEDICATION (PRODUCT NAME IN PARENTHESES)	DOSAGES IN MILLIGRAMS (TABLETS UNLESS OTHERWISE NOTED)	TYPICAL TREATMENT REGIMENS	POTENTIAL SIDE EFFECTS	INDICATIONS FOR USAGE (ITALICS = APPROVED BY U.S. FDA)
Venlafaxine (Effexor, Effexor XR)	25, 37.5, 50, 75, 100, 150, 225; XR 37.5, 75, 150	25–75mg twice per day (may be different for extended release)	Nausea, headache, insomnia, vivid dreams, sedation, jitteriness, dry mouth, constipation, diminished libido	*Depression*, anxiety
TRICYCLIC AND RELATED COMPOUNDS				
Amitriptyline (Elavil)	10, 25, 50, 75, 100, 150	10–50mg nightly	Confusion, forgetfulness, hallucinations, light-headedness, blurry vision, urinary retention, dry mouth	*Depression*, anxiety
Imipramine (Tofranil, Tofranil PM)	10, 25, 50; PM 75, 100, 125, 150	10–50mg nightly; PM 100mg max in elderly	Same as above	*Depression*, anxiety
Nortriptyline (Pamelor)	10, 25, 50, 75mg capsules; 10mg/5ml solution	10–50mg nightly	Same as above	*Depression*, anxiety
Trazodone (Desyrel, Oleptro) also a serotonin modulator	50, 150, 300	75–300 mg daily (divided)	Same as above	*Depression*, anxiety
OTHER ANTIDEPRESSANTS				
Bupropion (Wellbutrin, Wellbutrin SR, Wellbutrin XL, Budeprion SR, Budeprion XL, Zyban)	75, 100; SR 100, 150, 200; XL 150, 300	75–150mg 1–2 times daily (may be different for extended release)	Dry mouth, insomnia, headache, nausea, constipation, weight neutral, lack of sexual side effects, lowers seizure threshold	*Depression*

MEDICATION (PRODUCT NAME IN PARENTHESES)	DOSAGES IN MILLIGRAMS (TABLETS UNLESS OTHERWISE NOTED)	TYPICAL TREATMENT REGIMENS	POTENTIAL SIDE EFFECTS	INDICATIONS FOR USAGE (ITALICS = APPROVED BY U.S. FDA)
Mirtazapine (Remeron, Remeron SolTab)	7.5, 15, 30, 45; regular or orally disintegrating tablets	15–30mg daily	Drowsiness, increased appetite, headache, vivid dreams, lack of sexual side effects	Same as above; also available in orally disintegrating form
BENZODIAZEPINES				
Alprazolam (Xanax, Xanax XR, Niravam)	0.25, 0.5, 1, 2, 3mg tablets; 1mg/ml solution; XR 0.5, 1, 2, 3	0.25–1mg 3 to 4 times daily (may be different for extended release)	Drowsiness, light-headedness, depression, headache, confusion, dizziness, fatigue, constipation, blurred vision	*Anxiety/panic*; also available in orally disintegrating form
Clonazepam (Klonopin)	0.125, 0.25, 0.5, 1, 2	0.25–2mg up to 3 times daily	Same as above	*Anxiety/panic*; also available in orally disintegrating form
Diazepam (Valium)	2, 5, 10mg tablets; 5mg/5ml solution	1–5mg up to 4 times daily	Same as above	*Anxiety/panic*
Lorazepam (Ativan)	0.5, 1, 2mg tablets; 2mg/ml concentrate	0.5–2mg up to 3 times daily	Same as above	*Anxiety/panic*
OTHER ANTI-ANXIETY MEDICATIONS				
Buspirone (BuSpar)	5, 7.5, 10, 15, 30	5–15mg twice per day	Dizziness, drowsiness, dry mouth, nausea, headache	Generalized *anxiety* disorder
Propranolol (Inderal, Inderal LA, InnoPran XL)	10, 20, 40, 60, 80mg tablets; 20mg/5ml & 40mg/5ml solution; LA 60, 80, 120, 160; XL 80, 120	10–40mg up to 3 times daily (may be different for extended release)	Decreased heart rate, depression, exacerbation of preexisting asthma	Anxiety/panic (can suppress outward signs, such as racing heartbeat and shakiness)

Anxiety

Anxiety has been described by many experts as excessive worry about negative outcomes or events. A little anxiety can help a person plan and use caution to avoid dangerous situations; however, when anxiety is excessive, it can interfere with enjoyment and detract from daily function. About one in three people with Parkinson's disease meet the criteria for at least one type of anxiety disorder, with some studies finding the numbers even higher, up to 60 percent. Some anxiety can be generalized (it is experienced across many different areas of life), whereas social anxiety refers to being in social settings and may involve concern over the perception of others within these settings. Social anxiety is observed at all stages of Parkinson's disease, sometimes even before obvious symptoms emerge.

SYMPTOMS OF ANXIETY

- Being overly worried or apprehensive
- High levels of anticipation or being too focused on the details of a situation
- Being emotionally unstable or reactive
- Being overly fearful or avoidant
- Inability to stop thinking about something (rumination)
- Having many physical complaints

It is also important to keep in mind that anxiety on its own does not have the following symptoms (but these could occur if anxiety co-exists with depression):

- Experiencing lack of interest
- Experiencing morbid (dark doom and gloom) thinking
- Having feelings of guilt
- Having persistent feelings of sadness
- Experiencing loss of self-confidence or self-worth

Causes of Anxiety in Parkinson's Disease

The causes of anxiety in Parkinson's disease can be related to chemical neurotransmitter systems and to changes in levels of dopamine, serotonin, noradrenaline, and gamma aminobutyric acid (GABA). Anxiety is therefore a biological problem that can be related to Parkinson's disease. Even if medication for Parkinson's disease is regulated, anxiety may persist and require intervention. Anxiety can be compounded by a legitimate worry over life circumstances, as is the case in depression. Furthermore, anxiety can also be a symptom of the wearing off of Parkinson's disease medication. Deciding which of these factors most significantly contributes to a patient's anxiety is important to help find the most effective management strategy. For example, if the anxiety is episodic and occurs up to 30 minutes before the next dose of Parkinson's disease medication is due, it may be a symptom of the medication wearing off and a possible strategy would be to shorten the length of time between taking medication.

Motor symptoms, like tremor reemergence or muscle cramps, can be indicators that medication is wearing off, but anxiety can also be a wearing-off symptom. Some sufferers will describe feeling an "internal tremor" or a more distinct sense of panic or distress that settles down after the next dose of dopamine takes effect. When anxiety is consistent across the day, independent of medication timing, it may need to be addressed with therapy or medications. Some of the same treatments that are effective for depression may be useful for anxiety.

It is important to have a mental health professional make the correct diagnosis of possible anxiety disorders, including:

- Panic disorder
- Phobias (fears)
- Generalized anxiety disorder
- Social phobia (fear)
- Agoraphobia (fear of crowds)
- Post-traumatic stress disorder
- Anxiety disorder (not otherwise or specifically classified)

Penelope is a 59-year-old woman diagnosed with Parkinson's disease at age 51. She had been doing well with her medication (Sinemet 25/100, $1\frac{1}{2}$ pills, every four hours) over the past year. Recently, 30 minutes before her next dose of medication is due, she has been feeling nervous and jittery. She reports the anxious feeling to be very bothersome and she cannot easily explain what she is feeling.

Penelope is experiencing "off period anxiety." While some Parkinson's patients notice the reemergence of tremor when their medication wears off, others experience non-motor symptoms, such as anxiety. Her neurologist offers her a few options. One is to change her medication schedule to taking it every $3\frac{1}{2}$ hours to help avoid the wearing-off effect. Other options are to try longer-acting levodopa or to add adjunctive (helper) medication to try to extend the duration of each dose. In Penelope's case, adding entacapone to each dose helps extend the "ON" periods and avoid the wearing-off anxiety.

Treatments for Anxiety in Parkinson's Disease

There are a number of treatments for anxiety in Parkinson's disease. Here are some of the most common.

Cognitive Behavioral Therapy (CBT)

CBT can be performed in individual or group settings and can be helpful in planning for anxiety about future symptoms and also reactions to current changes and/or losses in life events. The goal of CBT should be to help maximize function within the current life situation. It is ideal if the therapist has familiarity with Parkinson's disease, but that may not always be available.

Selective Serotonin Reuptake Inhibitors (SSRIs) and Tricyclic Antidepressants

SSRI medications work to boost serotonin. The same considerations that were discussed relating to their use in treating depression also apply to their use in treating anxiety.

Buspirone

This medication is a little different from the medications utilized for depression. It has an impact on both serotonin and dopamine levels. It has a short duration of action, so must be taken two to three times daily.

Benzodiazepines

These medications help "tranquilize" anxiety by enhancing the calming effect. They block the chemical neurotransmitter GABA. These drugs are very sedating, however, and increase the risk of falling. They are also commonly reported as causing sleepiness and confusion. Most importantly, they do not correct or address the underlying serotonin imbalance, but instead help manage the symptom of the problem by increasing sedation and reducing anxiety. Although benzodiazepines can be helpful in specific situations, the help of a treating psychiatrist is often required to manage them.

Cannabinoids

There are cannabinoid receptors throughout the brain and there is emerging research that cannabidiol (CBD) oil and medical marijuana may be powerful treatments for anxiety, pain, and sleep dysfunction in Parkinson's disease. One caution is that benefits and side effects are not yet clear and patients taking cannabinoids may be at higher risk for side effects, including more automobile accidents. In our practice, we recommend that CBD formulations without THC should be utilized before recommending low-THC products. This approach seems to be less sedating and have fewer neuropsychiatric side effects.

→ **CLINICAL PEARL**

Anxiety, like other non-motor symptoms in Parkinson's disease, has to be screened for and addressed, as the balance in brain chemicals and the symptoms could change, requiring a change in treatment. Make sure you understand if your anxiety is generalized (meaning, it is there all the time) or if it is a result of the wearing off of Parkinson's disease medications. The former is more difficult to treat and will likely require a psychiatrist, and the latter can be addressed by moving dosages of dopamine closer together.

Apathy

Apathy is important to understand and to address; however, treatment options are still not clearly established. Some people with Parkinson's disease report a loss of motivation (which is due to changes in brain circuits) or a care partner might notice decreased initiative or interest in activities or engaging in conversation. In some cases, there is a decrease in the interest about the feelings of a care partner (what some experts refer to as "emotional indifference"). About half of the time, apathy occurs without depression or memory changes, and in those cases, it can be difficult to know what to treat, as depression and/or thinking problems may be targeted by medications. Many studies suggest that changes in dopamine circuits and depletion of dopamine may be part of the problem, and some imaging studies have suggested that degeneration in the front of the brain is important to the emergence of apathy.

APATHY AND DEEP BRAIN STIMULATION (DBS)

It is important to keep in mind that apathy may follow DBS treatment. This type of apathy may arise or become intensified by overaggressive reduction in medication following the surgical procedure. The reinstitution of dopaminergics may be a useful treatment.

Strategies to Address Apathy

Many medications have been used to address apathy, including dopamine agonists, MAO inhibitors, rivastigmine, antidepressants, stimulants, and anticholinergics. Rivastigmine revealed benefit in one small study. Cognitive training, exercise, and social engagement have also been recommended. Of all the medical treatments for apathy, dopamine agonists have been the most effective, but have also had the most side effects. If a dopamine agonist is administered, the care partner and family must be engaged to monitor for impulse control and other behavioral disorders.

In our experience, social activity is very important, both for people with Parkinson's disease and for care partners and family. One approach is to schedule activities and to work with care partners to execute activities at exact times and on specific days. Planning to exercise "when I feel like it" is less effective than "I will go with my care partner Monday, Wednesday, and Friday at 2 p.m." Day-to-day fluctuations in Parkinson's disease symptoms occur, and it is important to recognize that some unpredictable adjustments may need to be made for "good days" and for "bad days." Scheduling activities can facilitate overcoming the obstacle of apathy.

Other habits that can help manage apathy include:

- Scheduling activities, even if there is no desire to take part at the time of scheduling.
- Modifying activities as an alternative to eliminating them (e.g., golf fewer holes instead of stopping the hobby altogether).
- Having a buddy for each activity and encouraging each other to show up.
- Planning activities around medication timing if needed to optimize performance.
- Getting rest and maintaining a healthy, balanced diet. Exhaustion can only compound apathy.
- Taking it slow and allowing time for breaks.
- Taking note of the activities a person enjoys or has enjoyed in the past and making sure they are a regular part of life.

Apathy and Depression

When apathy is accompanied by a loss of enjoyment (referred to by experts as "anhedonia") as well as a diminished mood, it may be a sign of depression. Changes in energy and appetite can occur from Parkinson's disease (even without depression) and these symptoms can be difficult to separate from apathy and depression. Other signs of depression include having feelings of guilt and hopelessness. When apathy is associated with depression, it is important to seek treatment.

MORE APPROACHES TO TREATING APATHY IN PARKINSON'S DISEASE

London Butterfield and Dawn Bowers at the University of Florida developed the Parkinson's Active Living Program (PAL) specifically to address apathy. The program is primarily telephone-based and involves six weeks of scheduling activity and monitoring intervention to reduce levels of apathy.

Another approach is to listen to audiobooks along with a care partner, one chapter at a time, then stop after each chapter to have a discussion about it. If both decide together that they have comprehended the concepts of the chapter, proceed to the next. If not, repeat the previous chapter. This is also a potential treatment for cognitive dysfunction that is practical and enjoyable.

Demoralization

One important aspect of Parkinson's disease to recognize is that one in five patients become demoralized, and demoralization may not always be accompanied by depression, anxiety, or a mood disorder. Recognizing demoralization is important because Parkinson's disease can decline quickly once a patient "gives up." In such cases, we aggressively treat depression, apathy, fatigue, and sleep issues. We also use neuropsychology, psychiatry, and admission to the rehabilitation hospital for seven to 10 days, as appropriate. Although there is very limited data available, we find the multidisciplinary inpatient approach to be the strongest approach to treat demoralization.

Fatigue

One of the most common and most disabling symptoms in Parkinson's disease is fatigue. There are many factors that may contribute to fatigue, and teasing the factors apart can help determine what interventions may be helpful. Before attributing fatigue solely to Parkinson's disease, it is important to evaluate for general health conditions, like underactive thyroid, anemia, or diabetes. These and other health conditions can have an impact on energy level. Fatigue can be a primary symptom of Parkinson's disease, but it can also result from related, co-occurring symptoms, such as sleep dysfunction.

Medication can also be a common source of fatigue. Most of the medications used for Parkinson's disease, as well as many of those used for other general medical conditions, can result in tiredness. When Parkinson's disease medications wear off between doses, some people report feeling less energy or a decrease in endurance. A common complaint is leg or upper thigh weakness.

Fatigue and sleepiness are considered together by some experts. Sleep disorders are very common in Parkinson's disease, and insufficient or ineffective sleep can be part of the problem. A doctor can help screen for these types of problems by asking questions about movement during sleep, snoring, and frequent awakening. A sleep study may also be ordered to help assess for treatable disorders of sleep. When quality of sleep is improved, daytime energy may also improve. Waking at night to urinate is another common problem leading to daytime sleepiness. This problem may be assessed with medication and other strategies (see Chapter 5).

DID YOU KNOW?

One in three people with Parkinson's disease consider fatigue to be their most disabling symptom.

Avoiding "Deconditioning"

It is useful for patients to keep in mind the old adage "use it or lose it" in their approach to remaining active, because decreasing exercise can contribute to poor endurance, making it challenging to sustain a level of activity. When deconditioning is a concern, a supervised rehabilitative exercise program, such as working with physical and occupational therapies, may be advisable. Depression may cause fatigue, and if present, treating depression is the first appropriate step. Sometimes, fatigue is simply part of Parkinson's disease and may be caused by changes in brain circuits and not explainable simply by depression, sleep issues, or medication. There is very limited scientific evidence supporting a specific medication for the treatment of fatigue; however, rasagiline and doxepin have been suggested as possibilities. Interestingly, caffeine and stimulant medicines like methylphenidate and modafinil have not been shown to be effective.

MEDICATIONS AND FATIGUE

The following medications may result in fatigue for patients with Parkinson's disease:

◆ Narcotics (hydrocodone, oxycodone, morphine)

◆ Analgesics (other pain relievers)

◆ Muscle relaxants (cyclobenzaprine, tizanidine, baclofen)

◆ Benzodiazepines (alprazolam, lorazepam, clonazepam)

◆ Sedatives and sleep aids (diphenhydramine, zolpidem)

◆ Other antihistamines for allergies (hydroxyzine)

◆ Anticonvulsants used for pain (gabapentin, pregabalin)

◆ Some antidepressants (mirtazapine, amitriptyline, nortriptyline)

◆ Dopamine agonists (pramipexole, ropinirole, rotigotine)

◆ Higher-dose levodopa

Cognitive Changes

Memory and cognitive (thinking) issues may be areas of concern for some people with Parkinson's disease, and can range from having no impact to mild forgetfulness and word-finding trouble to significant and severe memory problems. In cases where "thinking" issues have an impact on daily life, there are some treatments available.

One of the most common thinking issues people with Parkinson's disease can experience is known as "executive

IS PARKINSON'S DISEASE THE SAME AS ALZHEIMER'S DISEASE?

No! Parkinson's disease and Alzheimer's disease are two different conditions, with tissue changes and changes in the brain that are different. Most Parkinson's disease patients with cognitive symptoms, when undergoing formal neurocognitive testing, will have a different pattern of results when compared to those with Alzheimer's disease. It is also possible for a person to develop both conditions, particularly as the risk for both increases with age.

dysfunction," which has been described as having trouble with planning and carrying out effective daily and work tasks. For instance, a person may have more trouble multitasking or may find it more difficult to manage attention, or to shift from one subject to another.

Another common cognitive complaint is trouble with word-finding or getting the words out of the mouth. We call this the "tip of the tongue" phenomenon and textbooks refer to it as a problem with verbal fluency. This type of problem, similar to memory issues, may involve changes in chemical neurotransmitter circuits that are not dopamine-dependent. As a consequence, when Parkinson's disease dopaminergic medications are successful for the visible movement problems, these types of cognitive difficulties can persist.

Studies have shown that some memory/cognitive medications may be mildly helpful in treating memory issues and are usually well-tolerated. These memory medications may be more helpful in Parkinson's disease memory issues than in Alzheimer's. The decision to use a memory medication should take into account the financial cost, pill burden, and whether the benefits of the medication outweighs the risks for the individual.

Causes of Cognitive Issues in Parkinson's Disease

Thinking and multitasking issues emerge from changes in the circuits involving the deep brain areas called the "basal ganglia" and also commonly from involvement of the frontal lobes. Since these changes are related to issues in the dopamine circuits, medications that help Parkinson's disease motor symptoms occasionally help thinking issues. It is not uncommon for those with Parkinson's disease to experience thinking issues (along with the reemergence of movement issues) with the "wearing off" of medication.

Mild Cognitive Impairment (MCI)

Mild cognitive impairment is a term that refers to experiencing memory or thinking issues that are mild and usually do not interfere with independent functioning. An example of MCI would be a person noticing that they are becoming a bit forgetful, but still managing to get the bills paid consistently and meeting all work expectations. MCI is not defined by a single description and is best diagnosed by a neuropsychologist who will perform a battery of tests and use standardized criteria.

Simple strategies, like keeping a calendar and adhering to a stable schedule, can be helpful when memory is a problematic symptom. For remembering medications, pillboxes can help provide visual confirmation that dosages have been taken, and alarms can function as reminders to take multiple doses. Although many people find cellular phone alarms to be useful, watches and pillboxes with alarms are also available. The most important factor for these

WHAT COGNITIVE/THINKING SYMPTOMS OCCUR IN PARKINSON'S DISEASE?

◆ Slowness of thought (bradyphrenia)

◆ Forgetfulness (memory impairment)

◆ Word-finding or verbal fluency issues ("It's on the tip of my tongue!")

◆ Trouble multitasking (working memory)

◆ Trouble planning and managing tasks (executive dysfunction)

◆ Visuospatial processing issues (understanding and processing pictures and objects in the environment)

strategies to work is committing to taking the medication immediately after hearing the reminder or alert.

For mild cognitive impairment, the best strategies include maintaining and enhancing physical, social, and cognitive activity. Physical exercise has been shown to assist in overall cognition, processing speed, and attention in Parkinson's disease. A 2018 study published in *PLoS One* showed that intense exercise has cognitive benefits. As the most effective approaches in regard to type and quantity of exercise are being studied, at present, an approach to exercise should be considered individually, based on an individual's capabilities, and safety should be the number-one priority. It is also useful to keep in mind that the best exercise is exercise that is enjoyed and performed consistently.

Parkinson's Disease and Dementia

When a person has severe cognitive symptoms interfering with daily or work activities, the term "dementia" is sometimes used to refer to this condition. Persons with Parkinson's disease should not panic if they experience these symptoms, nor mistake these symptoms for Alzheimer's disease. The most reasonable course of action is to be tested by a neuropsychologist, followed by a neurologist, and institute medications and/or behavioral treatments.

There is an increased risk for dementia in Parkinson's

→ CLINICAL PEARL

Depression can mimic dementia and, in some cases, the formal neuropsychological testing can conclude that a person actually has depression. When this occurs, experts refer to this condition as "pseudodementia." Treatment of depression and repeat neuropsychological testing can clarify the situation. Occasionally, a medication (e.g., a pain medication or sedative) can also mimic dementia in formal neuropsychological testing.

disease. Although experts have estimated this risk to be approximately five to six times the risk in the general population, these data can be misleading. Sometimes the dementia is due to memory loss related solely to Parkinson's disease, but in other cases, there may be strokes, Alzheimer's, or other conditions affecting the population being studied. It is important to not assume that all memory loss and thinking issues are due to Parkinson's disease alone, as there can be an overlap of conditions within the same individual.

Medications and Memory Difficulties

Prior to adding a medication to treat memory difficulties, it is important for a doctor to carefully review all medications that a patient is already taking. Many medications utilized for common issues, such as urinary urgency, may inadvertently result in confusion and thinking problems. Amantadine, dopamine agonists, and anticholinergic medications are common contributors to memory and thinking problems, and these medications may need to be adjusted or discontinued if thinking problems emerge. Other metabolic and nutritional issues should also be addressed, if present, and sleep should be optimized. Sleep deprivation can diminish thinking and memory in Parkinson's disease.

When all possible reversible factors have been addressed and behaviors (e.g., sleep) modified, the medications in the list that follows may be considered. The first three—rivastigmine, donepezil, and galantamine—are "cholinesterase inhibitors" (they enhance the activity of the chemical acetylcholine in the brain, which plays a major role in memory circuits). As they all have similar actions on the brain, they should not be administered together (choose only one if using this class of medication).

There are few side effects. The side effects we have commonly encountered over the years include nausea, diarrhea, and confusion. The last medication in this list, memantine, is thought to act on a different chemical (glutamate) and in our practice has been less well tolerated by many of our Parkinson's disease patients and can sometimes lead to worsened confusion or thinking.

Rivastigmine

This medication has U.S. FDA approval specifically for mild to moderate dementia in Parkinson's disease. It is available in capsule form and taken twice daily with food, or it can be administered in patch form.

Donepezil

This medication does not have U.S. FDA approval specifically for the treatment of Parkinson's disease. It is commonly utilized for mild to severe memory/thinking problems and its use has been based on its approval for treatment of Alzheimer's disease. Many neurologists, based on shown benefits, consider donepezil more effective for Parkinson's disease than for Alzheimer's disease (a safe dosage is usually to take it once daily).

IMPORTANT CONSIDERATIONS IN THE EVALUATION OF MEMORY AND COGNITIVE ISSUES

◆ Make sure depression is not clouding and confusing the perception of memory and thinking issues.

◆ Check the medication list to be sure drugs intended for specific purposes (bladder drugs, sleep aids, pain medications) are not resulting in memory and thinking issues.

◆ Optimize sleep.

◆ Identify and treat urinary tract infections (may be present without urinary symptoms).

◆ Watch out for amantadine, dopamine agonists, and anticholinergics (e.g., Benadryl/trihexyphenidyl).

DELIRIUM VERSUS DEMENTIA

Delirium has been described as a sudden state of confusion, often with fluctuating alertness. Delirium is typically provoked by a change in what experts refer to as "homeostasis" (the stable state of the mind and body). For example, homeostasis can be disrupted by an infection (most commonly a urinary infection), an imbalance in electrolytes (elements in the blood like sodium, potassium, calcium, and magnesium), or by a decline in kidney or liver function. Additionally, when a person is in the hospital, loss of sleep and being in an unknown environment can lead to delirium. When a sudden change in thinking or alertness is observed, the person suffering should be immediately evaluated, because in many cases there are reversible causes of delirium.

Dementia most commonly begins as a slower-onset condition with a progressive change in thinking that occurs over many years. In dementia, in many cases, alertness is largely preserved. People who have dementia may be more vulnerable to delirium when they experience imbalances, infections, or changes in their known environment. Dementia is diagnosed by a neuropsychologist or physician and can be followed and tracked by a neurologist.

Galantamine

Similar to donepezil, this medication is utilized "off label" (that is, not according to U.S. FDA approval) for treatment of dementia in Parkinson's disease. Galantamine is prescribed in immediate and extended release forms and is usually well-tolerated.

Memantine

This cognitive/thinking medication has a different mechanism of action than the previous cholinesterase inhibitors (it affects circuits related to glutamate rather than acetylcholine). The medication is available in short- and long-acting forms and it must be adjusted for people with kidney disease. The impact of memantine has been thought by most experts to be less than the impact of cholinesterase inhibitors, but it is often tried or added to a cholinesterase inhibitor.

Overall, medication for treatment of cognitive and thinking issues in Parkinson's disease may, in select cases, provide mild benefit. The medications are generally well-tolerated. If side effects occur, they are usually mild and may include tiredness, upset stomach, dizziness, or vivid dreams. The decision on whether to try one of these medications should be discussed with a treating physician who can generate a risk-benefit profile. We find it useful in our practice to obtain formal neuropsychological testing before treatment and to monitor with follow-up testing at intervals of six to 12 months. This strategy facilitates future discussions as to the long-term use of these medications for patients with Parkinson's disease and for cognitive/thinking issues.

→ CLINICAL PEARL

Most experts will start treatment with a cholinesterase inhibitor at least six to 12 weeks before considering the addition of memantine.

Cognitive Rehabilitation

There are many researchers engaged in the study of cognitive rehabilitation through the use of computers and video games. This area of research is founded on the principle that the brain is like a muscle, and if we exercise it, we can improve function. Although there has been very limited research in this area, it looks promising. Most experts agree that the old-fashioned concept of "use it or lose it" should apply to Parkinson's disease. It will be important for companies that have entered the market to show specific Parkinson's disease data that confirms or refutes the usefulness of their products. Finally, we have observed, as previously described in regards to the treatment of apathy, that the use of audiobooks and chapter discussions has a mildly positive affect on thinking and cognition. This technique has not been tested in a clinical trial.

Psychosis

Hallucinations or unnecessary suspiciousness (paranoia), also referred to as "psychosis," can occur in Parkinson's disease. Usually these types of symptoms emerge many years into the illness. The first step in addressing Parkinson's disease psychosis symptoms is to determine if the symptoms are disruptive, disabling, or decapacitating. Illusions (feeling that something entered and left the visual field) do not always require treatment. Mild hallucinations with the retention

CASE EXAMPLE   DIMITRA

Dimitra is a 73-year-old woman who was diagnosed with Parkinson's disease nine years ago. She has had gradual adjustments in her medication over time. These adjustments have allowed her to continue most things she enjoys. She reports that sometimes she thinks she sees a shadow pass by her in her peripheral vision at night. Usually she turns and realizes "my eyes were just playing tricks on me." Occasionally, she may see a pair of socks on the floor and mistake it for a mouse, but she recognizes the reality and shrugs it off. In this situation, she and her doctor decide that treatment is not necessary, as she does not find the problem distressing.

of insight (knowing the image is false) do not always require treatment.

There can also be delusions or beliefs that are not consistent with reality. Delusions may include false impressions of spousal infidelity, excessive or unfounded fear of theft, and general suspicion of a conspiracy. When hallucinations or delusions become bothersome, more frequent, or hard to separate from reality, treatment should be aggressively pursued. In mild hallucinations with retained insight and in cases of mild illusions, there is debate among experts on how aggressive to be with treatment.

When psychosis symptoms unfold suddenly, it is critical to rule out new infection or electrolyte imbalances. A simple urinary tract infection with no obvious urinary symptoms can result in a patient experiencing confusion and/or hallucinations. Addressing the underlying infection often leads to a return to normal cognition/thinking for the patient. Sleep deprivation can also induce confusion or hallucinations. Finally, there should be a review of medications, because many medications can provoke or aggravate psychosis. Common offenders include anticholinergics. An important step in addressing psychosis is removing medications that are non-essential and potentially causing the issue. Amantadine and dopamine agonists (pramipexole, ropinirole, rotigotine), as well as higher dosages of levodopa, may aggravate or provoke psychosis. It is critical for medications to be fine-tuned over time, since the balance can shift with aging, with disease progression, and with the unintended consequences of medication changes. Since even levodopa can be a contributor, dosing must be optimized.

Medications to Address Psychosis in Parkinson's Disease

Once reversible causes of psychosis are removed, medications would be the next consideration. Many of the medications used to control psychosis (neuroleptics or antipsychotics) block dopamine receptors. Blocking dopamine receptors, in practical terms, means reducing dopamine transmission in the brain and an aggravation of Parkinson's disease symptoms.

A STRATEGY FOR ADDRESSING MILD PSYCHOSIS

Discuss this strategy with a doctor to help determine which medications to stop or change in order to address mild psychosis:

First: Stop anticholinergics (like trihexyphenidyl or benztropine).

Second: Stop MAO-B inhibitors (selegiline, rasagiline).

Third: Stop amantadine.

Fourth: Stop dopamine agonists.

Fifth: Stop COMT inhibitors (like entacapone or tolcapone, or medications that contain them).

Finally: Check if levodopa can be reduced without worsening the motor symptoms. If not, then consider the risk-benefit profile for adding a psychosis drug.

Note that the above may not always be the correct sequence for an individual Parkinson's disease patient. The most important principle of this approach is to make one change at a time and to assess the result of each change. This approach aims to be sure that each change is helpful, and a doctor can assess the outcome related to a particular medication change.

In more severe cases, it may be necessary to stop all medications except levodopa, monitor for side effects, and employ a safety plan to avoid injury from falling or other complications that may occur from stopping medications. When more severe psychosis occurs, a Parkinson's disease patient may require 24/7 assistive care. In some cases, hospitalization may be necessary, although we try to avoid this scenario if possible.

Dopamine-blocking medications can worsen stiffness, tremors, and slowness. Some of the most potent neuroleptics (dopamine-blocking drugs) are not recommended in Parkinson's disease.

Neuroleptics carry a "black box warning," which means that they can increase mortality, particularly in elderly patients suffering from dementia. Studies of patients with dementia placed on these medications showed an association with more deaths, typically from cardiovascular causes or infections. The exact relationship to the medications or to the severe disease state could not be completely established. It is important to keep in perspective that even Parkinson's disease patients who do not suffer from dementia have an increased risk of side effects and a higher mortality while on antipsychotic medication. Fortunately, newer drugs, called "atypical" neuroleptics (such as quetiapine), seem to be safer than the older or "first generation" neuroleptics (such as haloperidol).

The decision to initiate Parkinson's disease medication must consider how much the hallucinations or delusions are having an impact on wellness and safety for an individual patient. We know that these symptoms can be very disruptive to people with Parkinson's disease and to their caregivers. Commonly, a low dose of these medications may be required to improve quality of life and to help people remain at home. A decision to treat the psychosis must consider many factors. This decision should be made with the guidance of a treating physician familiar with the patient and the family and, preferably, with expertise in Parkinson's disease.

Fortunately, there are several options for medications to treat Parkinson's disease psychosis. The following options, unlike the older typical dopamine blockers (typical neuroleptics), can control symptoms without worsening Parkinson's disease motor symptoms.

Quetiapine

Quetiapine is the most commonly prescribed medication for Parkinson's disease psychosis. It is typically taken one to two times per day. Most experts will initiate therapies with low dosages (e.g., 12.5mg at night) and will increase the dose depending on need. Common side effects include weight gain or tiredness, so many patients prefer taking quetiapine at bedtime. This strategy is especially helpful if the hallucinations are present at night. Since antipsychotics as a class of medicines have a "black box warning," it is important to discuss the risk-benefit profile with a doctor. The warning states that the risk could be due to antipsychotics or patient-related factors, and that the exact cause is often unknown. Doses of quetiapine should be started low and increased gradually until symptoms are adequately reduced. This strategy has the potential to improve quality of life and is considered reasonably safe. Although randomized studies of quetiapine have been disappointing, most experts agree that it is helpful in improving sleep quality and mild cases of psychosis.

AN IMPORTANT NOTE

Before administering a medication for psychosis, other health conditions (for example, liver trouble or severe kidney trouble) should be evaluated to determine a risk-benefit ratio for prescribing medication therapy. Safe and appropriate dosing may vary if other health conditions are present.

Pimavanserin

Pimavanserin is the only U.S. FDA-approved medication specifically for Parkinson's disease psychosis. Pimavanserin is interesting because it does not work primarily by blocking dopamine receptors. It has additional mechanisms of action, and the most important seems to be affecting serotonin pathways. The drug is designed to suppress mild to moderate psychosis without aggravating the Parkinson's disease motor symptoms. The dosage is once daily, in the morning, at 34mg. This medication is usually well-tolerated. It can take several weeks for the benefits to take effect, so it may be helpful to overlap with another medication during initial therapy. Many experts will start quetiapine first and then add pimavanserin, later trying to reduce or discontinue the quetiapine. Some experts will begin treatment with the quetiapine and monitor closely during the first few weeks of treatment. The question as to whether this drug can, in some cases, worsen psychosis has been raised; therefore, it is important to check in with a doctor frequently after initiating therapy.

Clozapine

Clozapine is the oldest but most effective drug for Parkinson's disease psychosis. However, it carries the risk of a rare but potentially serious side effect called "neutropenia" (or "agranulocytosis"), which means an unsafe lowering of white blood cells, which may diminish the body's ability to fight infection. The U.S. FDA requires all patients and their prescribing doctors, as well as pharmacies, to be enrolled in a registry to closely monitor bloodwork for the safety profile related to this medication. In the first six months on this medication, weekly blood tests are mandated and prescriptions can only be written one week at a time and after confirming the results of the blood tests. Following

---

WARNING!

Some antipsychotic medications can aggravate Parkinson's disease symptoms and should be avoided. For example, haloperidol may result in worsening of tremor and stiffness in a person with Parkinson's disease. Medications like haloperidol, when administered in the inpatient setting, can delay recovery and prolong hospitalizations.

six months of weekly monitoring, the tests can be reduced to every two weeks. Following one year of safe results, bloodwork and prescriptions can be reduced to monthly monitoring. In our practice, we follow approximately 50 patients actively with clozapine therapy and we find it to be the most effective medication treatment for Parkinson's disease psychosis. In severe cases of psychosis, we have found that it warrants the time and effort required for the extensive blood monitoring.

Rivastigmine

Rivastigmine is a memory medication referred to as a "cholinesterase inhibitor" and it works on brain circuits important to memory (and in areas that use a brain chemical called "acetylcholine"). This medication may reduce mild hallucinations in a select few individuals. Since it is relatively

---

CASE EXAMPLE / SOTIRIS

Sotiris is a 69-year-old man who was diagnosed with Parkinson's disease 12 years ago. He and his wife have noticed over the course of the past year that he would have "mild" hallucinations, including seeing children or small animals, but he would always be reassured when his wife told him they were not really there. More recently, though, he has had a harder time recognizing when something is a hallucination or not. This bothers him and causes him distress.

Sotiris talks with his doctor about the issue. He has been sleep-deprived because of frequent overnight urinary issues and watching TV or playing computer games late into the night. These issues were addressed, but in his case, the problem was not resolved. Sotiris and his doctor determine that he does not take unnecessary medications that may aggravate hallucinations and that his levodopa cannot be reduced without sacrificing control of his motor symptoms.

Together they discuss medication options, including risks and potential benefits. Sotiris and his wife decide on trying a low dose of quetiapine at bedtime. He start with 12.5mg nightly with only partial benefit. After increasing to 25mg, he has only rare hallucinations and his sleep improves.

Note: Neuroleptics (antipsychotics) should not be considered as a first option for simple insomnia. If hallucinations or delusions occur and cause distress or a safety concern, neuroleptics should be considered.

---

safe and may have additional cognitive benefits, it may be considered an option for cognitive issues.

A Concluding Note

Neuropsychiatric symptoms can have significant impact on quality of life and can lead to disruption for an otherwise happy and healthy Parkinson's disease patient. Identification and treatment of these behavioral issues has the potential to improve quality of life even more than treatment of the motor symptoms.

TREATMENT OF NEUROPSYCHIATRIC PARKINSON'S DISEASE SYMPTOMS

*I've discovered that as the years go by,
sometimes we are energized and enlightened
and sometimes we are demoralized and disheartened
to realize that in some situations our beginning is
our end and in others our end is our beginning.*
— MARTIN GUEVARA URBINA

➤ Demoralization occurs in one in five patients with Parkinson's disease, and in many cases it is not accompanied by depression.

➤ Take urgent action to address demoralization in Parkinson's disease. Addressing demoralization can be lifesaving.

➤ Depression is the largest unmet hurdle in the treatment of Parkinson's disease.

➤ The majority of patients with Parkinson's disease have untreated depression and/or anxiety.

➤ The specific type of antidepressant is less important than the adjustment of the dose to the appropriate level.

- Anxiety, sleep, and pain can be addressed with medications such as benzodiazepines, but also, more recently, by CBD and cannabis products.

- If you are started on an antidepressant, you should be seen soon after (e.g., one month) for close follow-up.

- A good night's sleep will give you a better chance at a great next day.

- Though some hallucinations may be benign, most require treatment or close monitoring.

- Metoclopramide, Phenergan, and Compazine are all common drugs administered for other medical reasons; however, these drugs will make Parkinson's disease symptoms worse.

- Clozapine, quetiapine, and pimavanserin are the three medications that can address hallucinations and psychosis without worsening Parkinson's disease symptoms.

- Fatigue may result from medications or cocktails of medications.

- Sleepiness can result from high dosages of Sinemet or Madopar.

- A sleep study may reveal the reason for underlying fatigue.

SELECTED REFERENCES

Da Silva FC, Iop RDR, de Oliveira LC, Boll AM, de Alvarenga JGS, Gutierres Filho PJB, de Melo LMAB, Xavier AJ, da Silva R. Effects of physical exercise programs on cognitive function in Parkinson's disease patients: a systematic review of randomized controlled trials of the last 10 years. *PLoS One*, 2018 Feb 27;13(2):e0193113.

Han JW, Ahn YD, Kim WS, et al. Psychiatric manifestation in patients with Parkinson's disease. *Journal of Korean Medical Science*, 2018;33(47):e300.

Mueller C, Rajkumar AP, Wan YM, Velayudhan L, Ffytche D, Chaudhuri KR, Aarsland D. Assessment and management of neuropsychiatric symptoms in Parkinson's disease. *CNS Drugs*, 2018 Jul;32(7):621–35.

Reijnders JS, Ehrt U, Weber WE, Aarsland D, Leentjens AF. A systematic review of prevalence studies of depression in Parkinson's disease. *Movement Disorders*, 2008 Jan 30;23(2):183–89; quiz 313.

Sawada H, Umemura A, Kohsaka M, Tomita S, Park K, Oeda T, Yamamoto K. Pharmacological interventions for anxiety in Parkinson's disease sufferers. *Expert Opinion on Pharmacotherapy*, 2018 Jul;19(10):1071–76.

Seppi K, Ray Chaudhuri K, Coelho M, Fox SH, Katzenschlager R, Perez Lloret S, Weintraub D, Sampaio C; and the collaborators of the Parkinson's Disease Update on Non-Motor Symptoms Study Group on behalf of the Movement Disorders Society Evidence-Based Medicine Committee. Update on treatments for nonmotor symptoms of Parkinson's disease: an evidence-based medicine review. *Movement Disorders*, 2019 Feb;34(2):180–98.

APPENDICES

"WHAT'S NEW IN PARKINSON'S DISEASE?"

ONE QUESTION WE commonly receive is: "What is the hope for the future of those with Parkinson's disease?" We believe the future should be balanced with excellent care, but also with the hope of cutting-edge therapies. These therapies will undoubtedly be revealed by advanced research.

We encourage all Parkinson's disease patients to engage in the research process and to enroll in clinical trials, and both patients and caregivers to become actively involved in the research process. The speed of new therapies will be directly related to the strength of the partnership with those afflicted with this disease. The path forward in Parkinson's disease will be lit by the hope that our children will not have to suffer.

As a final note, we would like to repeat one of the most important actions we have outlined in the pages of this book. Every Parkinson's disease patient and every caregiver should always ask one question at every clinical visit: "What's new in Parkinson's disease?"

FURTHER READING

Okun MS. *10 Breakthrough Therapies in Parkinson's Disease*. Books4Patients, 2015.

Okun MS. *Parkinson's Treatment: 10 Secrets to a Happier Life*. Books4Patients, 2013.

THE RESEARCH PROCESS

The research process begins with development of a new compound in the lab, continues with the three phases of clinical research, and concludes with approval by the U.S. Food and Drug Administration.

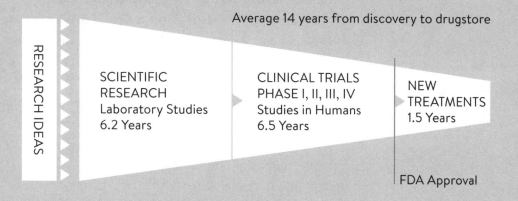

Average 14 years from discovery to drugstore

RESEARCH IDEAS

SCIENTIFIC
RESEARCH
Laboratory Studies
6.2 Years

CLINICAL TRIALS
PHASE I, II, III, IV
Studies in Humans
6.5 Years

NEW
TREATMENTS
1.5 Years

FDA Approval

This research process diagram is based on one developed by the Parkinson's Foundation educational series, and is presented with permission.

CARING FOR THE CAREGIVER

It is not the load that breaks you down.
It is the way you carry it.
– Lena Horne

STUDIES HAVE STRONGLY suggested that the most important factor for long-term success in Parkinson's disease is that the patient has a dedicated caregiver or care-partner. Unfortunately, the data also suggest that caregiver and care-partner strain occurs in the majority of families touched by Parkinson's disease. And, tragically, in most cases this strain goes unaddressed. Caregiver and care-partner strain have been shown to lead to worse outcomes, more emergency room visits, and more hospitalizations.

In our clinics, we advocate for self-care. If you are not well yourself, you will not be able to help others. If you have ever been on an airplane, you have likely heard the safety briefing that tells you that you must put on your own oxygen mask first, before you assist others. The same rule applies to caregivers and care-partners.

In our practice, at every visit with a patient with Parkinson's disease, we take the time to ask the caregiver or care-partner two questions:

"How are you doing?"

"Is there anything we can do to help you?"

We also always take time to show the patient and the family the data on the importance of the presence of an effective caregiver or care-partner, and to explain the importance of addressing caregiver or care-partner strain.

A Brief Guide for Caregivers

If you are caring for a person with Parkinson's disease, here is a checklist you can follow to help you with your task:

- Learn about Parkinson's disease from reliable sources and vet information through your doctor and care team.
- Verify all information that you get from the internet.
- Be wary of the fees charged for stem cell treatments or other potential cures.
- Be aware that each person with Parkinson's disease will be unique in their symptoms and lifespan, and that prediction is difficult with individual patients.
- Keep an updated list of medications and a list of doctors and contacts for the doctors and therapists. Keep these lists in your wallet and in the wallet of the person you are caring for.
- If deep brain stimulation (DBS) therapy is utilized, keep a bracelet or wallet card with information for care providers.
- If Duopa pump therapy is in use, prepare a wallet card or accompanying list of other pills.
- Keep a Parkinson's Foundation hospitalization kit handy, in case a hospital stay is needed.
- Make a list of your questions before doctor visits.
- Attend appointments together, as four ears are better than two.
- Consider detailed advanced planning (wills/advanced directives) and involve your doctors and care team in the discussions.

Additionally, we can offer a few more tips to help you support yourself, and to make sure you are in the best position to be able to provide care for others:

- If you don't have one already, find a sense of humor. Without one, you'll often despair. Find something funny in every day and in every moment. You need to laugh, as laughing is therapeutic.
- Don't beat yourself up. There will be good days and bad days. You may have more bad days than good days in your new unwanted role.

- If you notice changes in expression, motivation, and mood in the person you are caring for, remember that these can be part of Parkinson's disease and are not likely due to a diminishment in love.
- Don't focus all of your time on caretaking and disease management; do fun things that do not revolve around Parkinson's disease.
- You need your friends. Don't alienate them by trying to do this by yourself. Accept invitations to help. Accept an hour off, or an offer to pick up some groceries, drop the kids off at practice, or cook the family a meal. Give yourself some slack and let your friends feel needed and feel included.
- Try a support group, locally or even online. You may not think you need it, but you may. As the road becomes bumpier, it is nice to travel with others who know the way. Remember, though, that support groups do not work for everyone. Try them, but do not blame yourself if they don't work for you.
- Keep communication lines open with family members and friends. It's important to stay connected to the people who care.
- Recognize that you are only human. Allow yourself to experience all emotions that surface. These emotions may include both resentment and guilt, and these are normal and expected responses. Cycles of these emotions may repeat and reemerge.
- Get help immediately if you feel an urge to harm your relative, friend, or yourself.
- Find an outlet for expressing your thoughts and feelings. Some outlets may include talking with a friend, keeping a journal, or attending a caregiver support group.
- Seek help from a social worker or clinical psychologist. Caregivers and care-partners who do this, in our experience, do better.
- Couples counseling can also be helpful.
- Remember that depression and anxiety are legitimate medical conditions and are treatable.

- Address your own needs as well as the needs of the person you are caring for. Devote independent time for yourself.
- Make every day your best day.

As a final note, we would like to address the confusion we have encountered in families about who to approach for help. For severe depression, anxiety, or mood disorder in a caregiver or care-partner, a psychiatrist, neurologist, or general doctor can evaluate and potentially prescribe and monitor medications. Medications are required for caregivers and care-partners in some but not all cases. For counseling, you should seek a social worker or counseling psychologist and not a neuropsychologist. A neuropsychologist performs memory and cognitive testing but does not, in most cases, also perform counseling.

PEARLS FOR A BETTER LIFE: A COMPLETE LIST

THE REALITY OF disease-oriented and self-help books is that, while they are well-meaning, frequently they meet their end on a dusty bookshelf. That's why, at the end of every chapter in this book, we have offered a list of "pearls for a better life": a few simple, helpful, and easy-to-remember aphorisms, or brief truths, that you, as a patient or caregiver, can put in your pocket to help you absorb and act on the information we have presented.

To make it even easier for you to find these pearls when you need them, we have collected them all again here, at the back of the book. Come back to these last few pages and review these bits of wisdom whenever you need a refresher on what you have learned in these pages.

Chapter 1: Getting the Diagnosis Right

- The four words "You have Parkinson's disease" are not a death sentence.
- Know what you don't have. Parkinson's disease is not Alzheimer's disease, ALS (Lou Gehrig's), or a brain tumor.
- Parkinson's disease patients can possibly live 20, 30, 40, or more years following diagnosis.
- Parkinson's disease is not one disease. It is a group of symptoms, and the symptoms can vary widely from patient to patient.
- Know your Parkinson's disease subtype (tremor dominant, akinetic rigid, postural-instability gait disorder).

- After therapy optimization, many patients with Parkinson's disease will tell us their lives are more meaningful following a diagnosis.
- "Live as if you were to die tomorrow. Learn as if you were to live forever." — Mahatma Gandhi
- Try to keep your soul young and quivering right up to old age. — George Sand

Chapter 2: Exercise and Rehabilitation Therapy

- Not all physical, occupational, and speech/swallow therapy is equal.
- Exercise is like a drug for Parkinson's disease. Before there were drugs for Parkinson's disease, exercise was the key.
- Rehabilitation therapy (PT, OT, speech/swallow) can be more powerful than drug therapy alone.
- Exercise and rehabilitation therapies are now considered first-line therapy for Parkinson's disease.
- Be careful taking a prescription for PT, OT, and/or speech/swallow therapy to a therapist who is not trained in Parkinson's disease.
- Bad therapy is worse than no therapy.
- Occupational therapy is important for reintegrating back into society and back into life.
- Speech can be improved by therapy.
- If you cough when eating or drinking, you may be at risk for aspiration pneumonia, which is the leading cause of death in Parkinson's disease.
- Swallowing issues can also lead to aspiration pneumonia.
- There are therapies for improving swallowing and preventing aspiration pneumonia.
- Continuous booster therapy (weekly or bimonthly) is superior to burst therapy (e.g., six to eight weeks of intensive therapy, and then done). Spread your rehabilitation therapy visits over an entire year.

- Teach a spouse, friend, or personal trainer to direct your home therapy.
- "All you need is the plan, the road map, and the courage to press on to your destination." — Earl Nightingale

Chapter 3: To Start or Not Start Medications for Parkinson's Disease

- Do not fall victim to levodopa phobia.
- You will not "receive a medal" for delaying therapy.
- If Parkinson's disease symptoms are affecting your quality of life or resulting in disability, it is time to start medications.
- The hospital is a dangerous place for the Parkinson's disease patient. Every effort should be pursued to avoid hospitalization.
- If hospitalized, become your own advocate. You can order an "Aware in Care" hospitalization kit from the Parkinson's Foundation.
- "Start by doing what's necessary; then do what's possible; and suddenly you are doing the impossible." — Francis of Assisi

Chapter 4: Medication for Parkinson's Disease Motor Symptoms

- Take the amount of medication you need to control your symptoms.
- If you are just changing the dose and not the time intervals in Parkinson's disease, you are probably doing something wrong.
- MAO-B inhibitors (selegiline, zydis selegiline, rasagiline, Xadago) provide very mild symptomatic effects and are not replacements for dopamine agonists or dopamine replacement.
- MAO-B inhibitors have not been definitively proven to be neuroprotective or to slow clinical disease progression.

- One in five to six people who start a dopamine agonist will develop an impulse control disorder. Always have a spouse or friend monitor for impulse control disorders when starting a dopamine agonist.
- Levodopa (Sinemet), especially at high dosages, can, rarely, result in manic behavior (hyperactive state) and compulsive sexual behavior, including possible strange behaviors.
- Dopamine extenders, such as entacapone and Stalevo, may require reduction in other dopamine dosages to lessen the risk of dyskinesia.
- The Duopa dopamine pump is a gel form of dopamine that can be continuously infused into the small intestine. The most common side effects from the pump are related to issues with the tube.
- "I believe in prescription drugs. I believe in feeling better." — Denis Leary

Chapter 5: Medications for Non-Motor Parkinson's Disease Symptoms

- The non-motor symptoms are more disabling than the motor symptoms of Parkinson's disease (tremor, stiffness, slowness).
- Do not be embarrassed to take an antidepressant.
- Do not hesitate to identify and treat anxiety.
- Determine whether anxiety occurs when wearing off medications and consider changes in medication timing.
- Treatment of non-motor symptoms will in many cases improve motor symptoms.
- Apathy is more common than depression in Parkinson's disease.
- Dopamine agonists and counseling therapy could be helpful for apathy.
- Support from a licensed clinical social worker or counseling therapist has been shown to enhance the effects of medication.
- Treat constipation aggressively, as it has a huge impact on quality of life.

- Pain medications are a common offender for causing constipation.
- "Worry never robs tomorrow of its sorrow, it only saps today of its joy." — Leo Buscaglia

Chapter 6: Surgical Therapies for Parkinson's Disease

- When selecting a surgical team, experience matters.
- Not everyone should receive deep brain stimulation (DBS) or other surgical therapies.
- The best scenario you can hope for is to be evaluated by a DBS multidisciplinary team who "talk behind your back" and plan every aspect of your surgery and aftercare.
- DBS surgery is not one-size-fits-all, and the brain target, approach (unilateral versus bilateral), and staging (one procedure or several) can make the difference between success and failure.
- The DBS lead location cannot be determined by imaging alone (CT or MRI) but is also determined by programming.
- The most critical element of DBS outcome after proper selection is location, location, location (of the DBS lead). No amount of expert programming can make up for a misplaced DBS lead.
- Once an adequate DBS setting is chosen, there are usually minimal if any programming changes over time. This is in contrast to medications and other therapies, which are in constant flux following DBS surgery.
- More important than DBS programming is monitoring and treating the neuropsychiatric and other aspects of the Parkinson's disease.
- DBS surgery is not a cure.
- The symptoms most likely to improve with DBS are tremor, rigidity, bradykinesia, off time, on-off fluctuations, and dyskinesia.
- Walking, talking, and thinking are usually not improved by DBS surgery.

- The choice of DBS device should occur as the last step in the multidisciplinary discussion. The device choice should be tailored as much as possible to your individual needs.
- All devices, regardless of manufacturer, will work well if optimally placed within the brain.
- Though radiosurgery and focused ultrasound are "incisionless," a permanent hole is still placed in the brain.
- Radiosurgery and focused ultrasound are therapies directed at the target from outside the brain. These therapies do not use physiological guidance or microelectrode recording.
- Radiosurgery, focused ultrasound, or conventional lesion surgery (pallidotomy, thalamotomy, subthalamotomy) should not be performed on both sides of the brain.
- Radiosurgery (gamma knife) has delayed benefits and delayed side effects, and the radiation damage can slowly spread into unintended brain areas.
- Ultrasound therapy has fewer infections and fewer bleeds.
- Brain lesion therapy should not be performed on both sides of the brain as it can lead to irreversible talking and thinking problems.
- "I have made many mistakes myself; I have spoiled a hatful; the best surgeon, like the best general, is he who makes the fewest mistakes." — Sir Astley Paston Cooper

Chapter 7: Nutrition and the Microbiome

- There is increasing evidence that there is a gut-brain connection in Parkinson's disease.
- The common gastrointestinal bug *H. pylori* affects approximately half of the world's population, and it can affect absorption of Parkinson's disease medications.
- Early research has revealed the possibility that certain diets (e.g., the Mediterranean diet) may be helpful in prevention and treatment of degenerative diseases.

- Probiotics and other nutritional approaches are promising; however, their effects across the Parkinson's disease population remain unknown.
- Foods, especially those containing protein, can influence absorption of Parkinson's disease medications.
- The majority of people with Parkinson's disease do not need to change their diet to improve medication absorption.
- The most common strategy to improve medication absorption is to give your medications a half hour more head start before you eat.
- If you love wine or alcohol, the safest way to consume it is in small quantities — pouring just enough in the bottom of the glass to allow taste without impairment.
- "Our bodies are our gardens and our wills are our gardeners." — William Shakespeare

Chapter 8: Treatment of Neuropsychiatric Parkinson's Disease Symptoms

- Demoralization occurs in one in five patients with Parkinson's disease, and in many cases it is not accompanied by depression.
- Take urgent action to address demoralization in Parkinson's disease. Addressing demoralization can be lifesaving.
- Depression is the largest unmet hurdle in the treatment of Parkinson's disease.
- The majority of patients with Parkinson's disease have untreated depression and/or anxiety.
- The specific type of antidepressant is less important than the adjustment of the dose to the appropriate level.
- Anxiety, sleep, and pain can be addressed with medications such as benzodiazepines, but also, more recently, by CBD and cannabis products.
- If you are started on an antidepressant you should be seen soon after (e.g., one month) for close follow-up.

- A good night's sleep will give you a better chance at a great next day.
- Though some hallucinations may be benign, most require treatment or close monitoring.
- Metoclopramide, Phenergan, and Compazine are all common drugs administered for other medical reasons; however, these drugs will make Parkinson's disease symptoms worse.
- Clozapine, quetiapine, and pimavanserin are the three medications that can address hallucinations and psychosis without worsening Parkinson's disease symptoms.
- Fatigue may result from medications or cocktails of medications.
- Sleepiness can result from high dosages of Sinemet or Madopar.
- A sleep study may reveal the reason for underlying fatigue.
- "I've discovered that as the years go by, sometimes we are energized and enlightened and sometimes we are demoralized and disheartened to realize that in some situations our beginning is our end and in others our end is our beginning." — Martin Guevara Urbina

Library and Archives Canada Cataloguing in Publication

Title: Living with Parkinson's disease : a complete guide for patients and caregivers / Michael S. Okun, MD, Irene A. Malaty, MD, Wissam Deeb, MD.

Names: Okun, Michael S., author. | Malaty, Irene A., author. | Deeb, Wissam, author.

Identifiers: Canadiana 20200193503 | ISBN 9780778806721 (softcover)

Subjects: LCSH: Parkinson's disease—Popular works. | LCSH: Parkinson's disease—Treatment—Popular works.

Classification: LCC RC382 .O38 2020 | DDC 616.8/33—dc23

INDEX

hypotension (orthostatic), 24, 94, 131–35

I

impulse control disorder (ICD), 98, 101, 102–3, 117
Inbrija (inhaled levodopa), 114
insomnia, 94. *See also* sleep disorders
instability (postural). *See* balance
iron deficiency, 140
istradefylline, 106

L

language difficulties, 56–57, 214
laxatives, 123–25, 180–81
Lee Silverman voice treatment (LSVT), 53
lesion therapies. *See* ablative therapies
levodopa (L-dopa), 72–78, 88, 90–96, 108. *See also* dopamine; *specific combination forms*
  alternative forms, 95, 97, 114, 117
  in combination, 91–93, 95, 97, 109, 114
  controversy about, 73–75
  diet and, 184–85
  dosages, 92, 97
  and dyskinesia, 76–77, 78, 79, 94–95
  as early treatment, 78, 79
  as nausea cause, 89–90, 91–92, 93–94
  and peripheral decarboxylase inhibitors, 91–93
  research on, 74–80, 95–96
  and restless legs syndrome, 141
  side effects, 93–96, 98, 117
lubiprostone, 123

M

Madopar (benserazide + levodopa), 230
malnutrition, 181–82
MAO-B (monoamine oxidase B) inhibitors, 73, 88, 100, 103–4, 108, 110–11. *See also specific drugs*
  for depression, 199–200

effects, 104, 117
marijuana. *See* cannabinoids
mask effect, 20
medications, 88, 108–11, 242. *See also specific drugs, drug classes, and conditions*
  absorption of, 139
  choosing, 85–86, 89, 91, 112
  and cognitive issues, 141
  constipation-causing, 125, 146, 178
  effects, 70, 88, 113, 152
  as fatigue cause, 213, 220
  "half-life" of, 92
  information about, 87
  for motor symptoms, 85–117, 138, 242–43
  need for, 67–69, 71, 79
  for non-motor symptoms, 119–47, 243–44
  as Parkinsonism cause, 29–30
  as psychosis cause, 222, 223, 224
  and sleep, 137, 139
  supplements as, 70–71, 88
melatonin, 137, 138, 144
memantine, 217–18, 220
memory medications, 144–45, 214, 217–18, 220. *See also* cognitive issues
Metamucil (psyllium husk powder), 124, 180
methylcellulose, 124, 180
metoclopramide, 94, 124, 230, 247
microbiome, 187–89
micrographia, 20
midodrine, 132–33
mirabegron, 126, 127
motor fluctuations, 113, 115
mouth problems, 27, 58. *See also* drooling
Mucuna pruriens (velvet bean), 70
multiple system atrophy (MSA), 30
muscle pain, 26

N

naps, 136, 137